MI Dishes & More

A **30** D A Y G U I D E TOWARDS A BETTER, HEALTHIER, HAPPIER YOU

By

Amina Pankey

MI_Dishes & More: A 30 Day Guide Towards A Better, Healthier, Happier You

is a work by Amina Pankey based on her workout routine.

The information in this book is strictly informational,

and the author shall in no instance be held liable for any risks

associated with the use of the material in this book.

ISBN - 9781798042298

Published and printed in the United States of America.

Cover Design by Moses Dalton, Photography by Amina Touray

Edited by Sonya Jenkins.

Acknowledgements

Thank you, to my daughters, Cori and Bronx. Yes, they will ALWAYS come first. They are my force behind this book, and everything else I do.

Thank you, to all you amazing women who motivate me everyday to continue to share my life. Although I hear how inspiring I am on a daily basis, in reverse, I get inspired by you and your messages and comments. I also want you all to know that I SEE YOU, even if you've never gotten a reply or comment back.

Thank you, to the people who contributed to this project in such a huge way and without whom it would not have been possible to put it all together: My photographer Amina Touray, and my book designer Moses Dalton. I appreciate you guys for putting so much passion into this project and always being fun to work with and completely drama-free.

The fact that this book includes so many pictures was my idea from the jump. I wanted to create a visual book where the pictures speak equally as much as the literal part and where they can inspire, even if you don't read. Obviously we shot most of these pictures with a direct plan but thanks to my photographer Amina Touray we've managed to have an exact representation of my actual life. I am thankful for this collab!

Thank you, to my best friend, Nicole, who is the mastermind behind the set-up of this book. Because of her

I decided to not only write a recipe book, which was my original plan, but a complete lifestyle guide that includes more than just food for you all! It was something we talked about over coffee. I actually took on the ideas she shared and completed this book while keeping her input in the back of my mind! Love you, Nicole!

Thank you, also, to my other half, my twin sister Jazz, who helped me put together some of the awesome workouts throughout this book, especially since I got lost in the process a couple of times. I had to make sure I had professional help, and she was the one to call!

Thank you, to my Mommy and my sister, Sophie, for helping me with a few of these yummy recipes. Your ideas and add-ons made this way more versatile and interesting than it would have been without you! A few of my favorite dishes came from you, and especially Mom, who made me unafraid to improvise when it comes to cooking. That's how I came up with some of the most delicious dishes.

Thanks to my editor, Sonya Jenkins, who over the past two years has supported me in everything I've done and has always shown genuine love, not just to me, but my baby girls. We love you for it!

I also wanna thank all of the amazing Yogis whom I've never met, but who inspire me daily by sharing their practices, as well as the fitness instructors who have taught me. I follow you with a passion and learn from you everyday.

Peaceful Day   *Fun Day*

Med/Light Work Day   *Hard Work Day*

Introduction

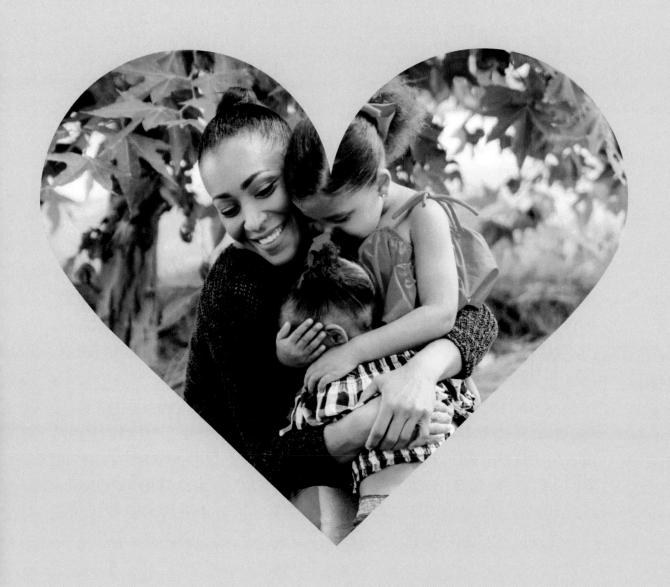

People always ask me how I do it all. They want to know how I balance life by being a mom, going after my dreams, pursuing my music career, working out on the regular, cooking for my kids and myself, keeping my kids entertained and happy, and on top of all that, looking good while doing so (most of the time😏).

Let me start by saying, It Ain't Easy. However, I decided to write this book because I've come up with a routine that helps me be happy and feel energized in my everyday, imperfect life. I have learned to balance everything that's important to me and feel good, while juggling all of those things better than ever, to be exact. I get messages every day from women asking me about the dishes I make, how I got into yoga or simply how I stay motivated and have such a positive energy around me. I want to share my little secrets with you!

Don't get me wrong, I don't always have it all together, I get overwhelmed and exhausted, and most days I fall into bed at night thinking, "How in the hell did I make it through the day again?" But the majority of my days now, compared to before, have me in a joyful and peaceful space that is absolutely priceless.

I believe the key to my success has been figuring out the things I need to do to make myself feel at ease, relaxed, and happy in the midst of the stressful life I live. In other words, I combat stress with activities and foods that give me the drive to continue a balanced and satisfying lifestyle.

Being a mom is stressful. If you are a mom (stay at home mom, working mom, single mom, whatever the case may be), you know how hectic it can get. You also know how exhausting it can be and how much the stress can drive us crazy. And we all certainly know the moments where we just simply need A BREAK! You can't go on and on, and keep going (nonstop) and not get to a point where you are worn out completely.

Despite the fact that we know this, it's not easy for many of us to take breaks. Time, money, and getting help all play a part in how we as moms, and women in general, can make these breaks possible. Besides that, it also is not easy for some to know HOW to take breaks correctly, so that they benefit you, give you energy, and recharge you physically and mentally. On top of all that, I even figured out some ways to include my children into my breaks. Yes, sounds crazy because when talking "breaks" one would think it would be necessary to be in a different space — alone, or at least away from the kids. But there are certain activities that you can do that focus on you, even with kids around. Kids do need to be trained a little when you're trying to do this, which I will go into a bit more later.

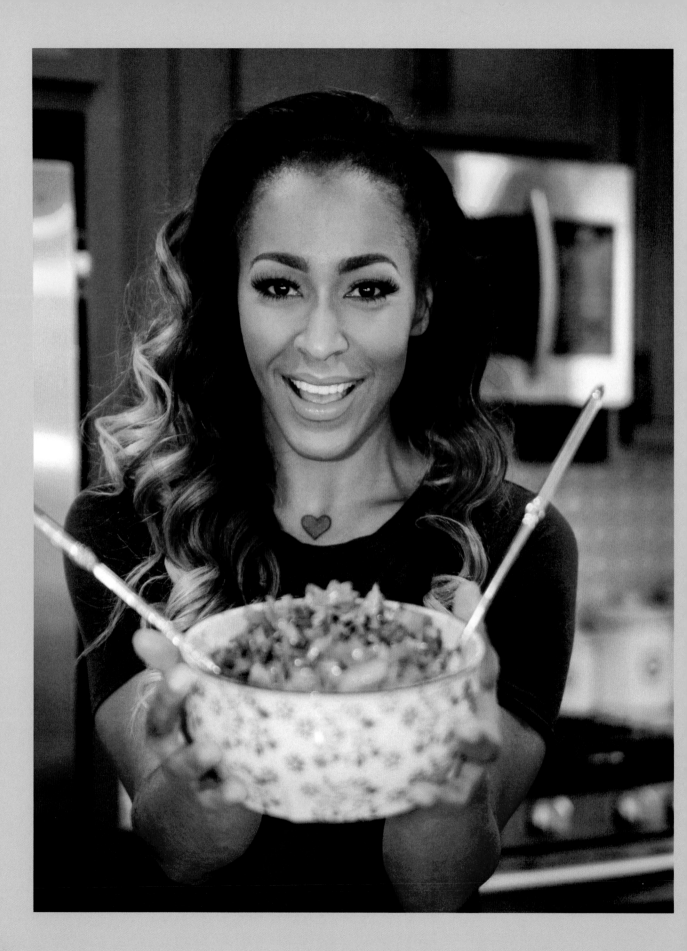

Being and staying in shape is so important to feeling good in the long run. Stuffing your face with junk food and being lazy also feels good, but the difference here is that it's temporary. It only feels good in the moment and while you're doing it. And being that it can have a negative effect on your overall well-being to just be lazy and eat all day, we should do it less! We still do it, but we keep it to a minimum. We focus on what makes us feel good for longer than just an hour or two.

So, you see, there are a lot of factors that are of value in this matter. I call them the Fs. They are what I spend most time and money on! And I don't ever regret it, because they are (and I've figured them out over time) what is so important to me and to my well-being.

Food

"You are what you eat." Everyone knows that saying. And it is very much true. What you put in your body can have an effect on not just your physical well being, but also your moods. It can have you feeling run-down or even depressed.

Being that I personally have no restrictions in my diet anymore (I used to ALWAYS diet before I had my kids), I've noticed what certain foods do to me during a certain time of the day. Whether it's positive or negative, the key here is balance. For example, if I have too big of a breakfast, my workout seems harder. Or, if I go to bed too hungry, it affects my sleep. Also, if I eat too much junk food all the time, my conscious won't stop beating me up about it. But if I have junk food sometimes, I've learned to accept and understand that it ain't a big deal. And I have learned to enjoy and appreciate those "bad foods" at a good time, even more … without the guilt.

Fitness

Physical challenge has always given me many benefits when it comes to feeling good. Not only do you feel better when you look better, but you also feel better when you master something difficult. In other words, it's good for your ego. Building strength, endurance and focus can be of amazing value for your overall well-being. Personally, I have always been into working out, but I used to hate working out and would only do it because it would help me maintain my figure, as well as make me feel good *afterwards*. Learning how to enjoy the "during" period of a workout — running, sweating, whatever it may be — and figuring out how to actually enjoy being active, was something that happened after I started YOGA. It is funny how a comparatively easy workout taught me to master the mind over matter mentality and apply that in my harder, more intense, high energy workouts, – by not thinking, but just DOING. Yogis may argue that

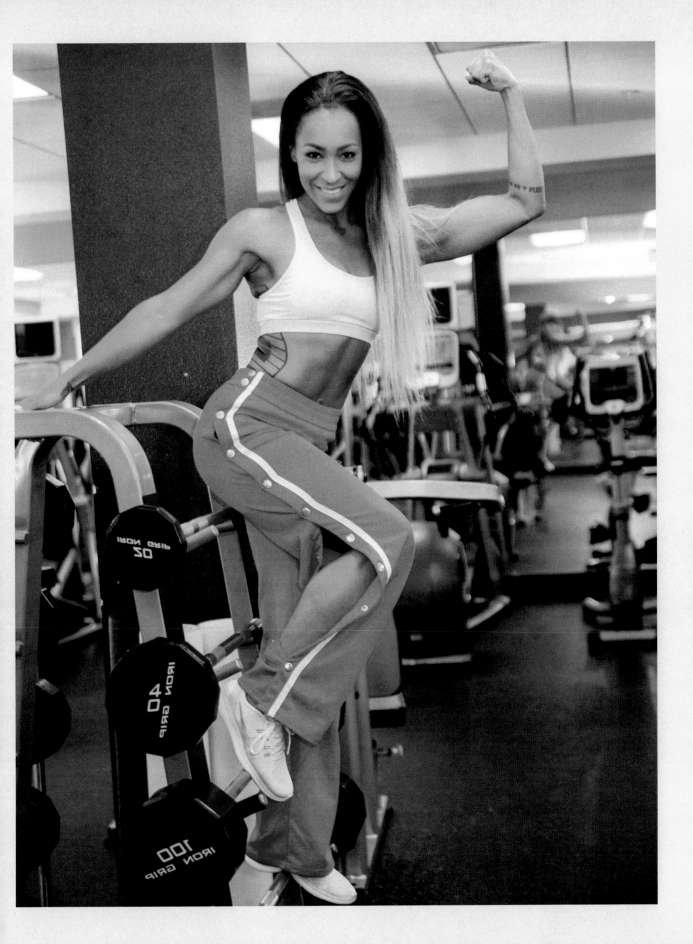

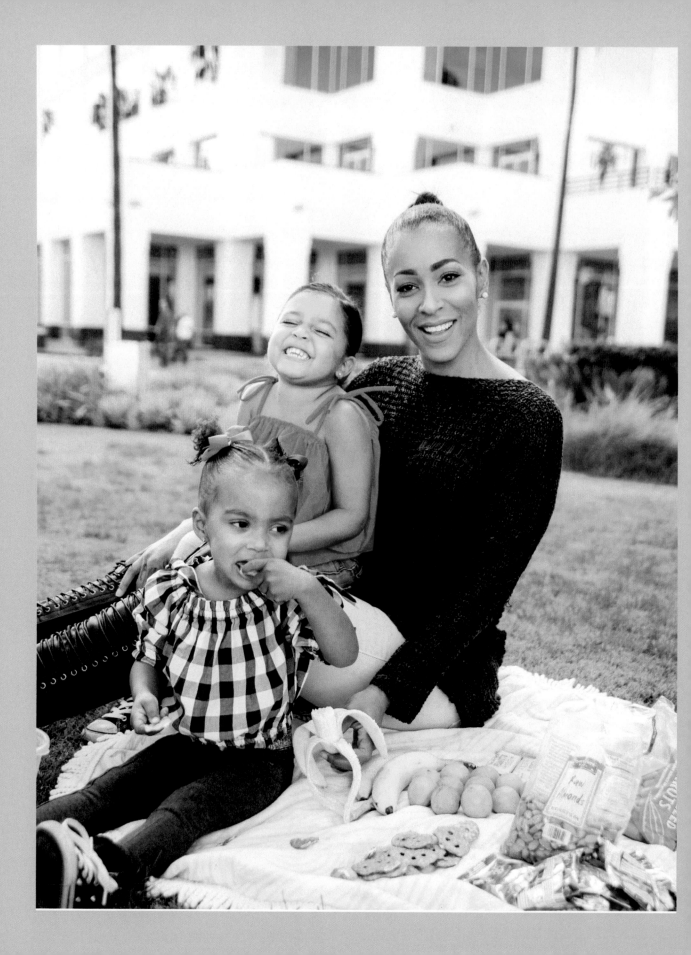

you cannot compare the two and I am not. Many won't even put YOGA into the box of a "workout," but to me it all goes together and it all fits under MY umbrella of FITNESS.

Fun

No time spent laughing is wasted time. Not until I was in my 30s was I able to have a good time playing without feeling guilty. I used to only feel happy if I had been productive or had worked towards my goals. I literally was living for something I hoped the future would bring, and so many others do this too. For me, it was a successful music career — the arrival at stardom. While I was getting there, I could not enjoy myself. I had to grow to learn that what matters is the MOMENT. The moment I have right now. And I had to have children to learn that *regular* things are not *regular* when you learn to appreciate them. Nowadays, I find so much joy in the simple things. Things like going for coffee or going to the park. I take it all in as if I were a child again. And thanks to my babies for that!! I needed to become a mom to go back to enjoying the simple things in life. Seeing how excited a child gets when he or she sees bubbles, clouds in the sky that form a shape, or going up in a transparent elevator just makes you go back to the moments when those things were new to you.

Doing something fun is so important, not only

because you make life worth living by being in the moment, but also for your inspiration, motivation and making memories, because memories last forever. Whatever it is that you like to do for fun, DO IT. Make time for it, especially when you work hard . . . Play Harder. My quality of life has risen since I realized this and it just keeps on rising.

Happiness is a FEELING inside of you. Many of us read quotes every day on how happiness is inside of us and not something that we get or find from another. When we truly realize this, everything becomes better. You become happier.

I personally have been in a place where I was ready to quit it all and I've also had those mood swings where one day I'm happy to be alive and the next day I want to just crawl under a rock. Overall, I can honestly say that today I am the happiest I have ever been - ALONE. Yes, I have my kids and they contribute to my happiness in a humongous way. They are the core of why I am a happier human and I always say that when asked how motherhood has affected me.

What I mean by ALONE is that I don't have a partner (at least not while writing this book). I am not rich, compared to a lot of people I'm surrounded by, and I do have my flaws — physical flaws, character flaws — we ALL got them. But as I once wrote in a song, "It's All Right": It's all right to be ordinary, It's all right that I'm not that rich and don't have this or that. It's all right to be a couple of steps behind what I want to be. You have to learn to be fine where you are while working towards making the necessary changes to reach your goals. It could always be better, but it could also always be worse. You're here, and you're alive. Don't wish for things to be easier, because most likely, they won't be easy. And if they are, another obstacle of life is waiting at the horizon. That's just how it is and that's something that can never be changed. Darker days just keep coming, but you can learn how to master a storm like a warrior. Work on yourself to become stronger, so that you are able to handle and deal with the difficulties life throws at you.

I want to help you feel better in your regular, everyday life because I've experienced being overwhelmed, feeling tired, feeling depressed and unmotivated so much in my life that I like to believe I've become a pro at "Getting myself out of a Funk," and especially because those low moments still happen and will continue to happen. There will always be ups and downs in life, but it is essential to know how to be okay in any kind of weather! Whatever you're going through, there is a way out, and I certainly may not have the answer to YOUR problems, but I believe I can help you feel a little more at ease, healthier and excited about life in general. We are going to be cooking, laughing, singing, dancing, hiking, running, sleeping, relaxing, shopping, driving, eating, drinking, talking, keeping silent, jumping, meditating, sweating, breathing (very important), and loads of other things.

With this guide, I am sharing workouts I do and dishes I like to eat that are probably 80 percent on the healthy side and 20 percent indulgence. I'm sharing exactly when and how often I have them, guiding you through 30 days in "My Style of Living." Again, what works for me may not work for you, but you can modify dishes and exercises. You can also switch around days as you please to accommodate your schedule. As long as you complete each day, you will master my guide. Great, ain't it? I have to mention that this is not a weightloss guide, but more-so a guide to a healthier, happier you. You may or may not lose weight. It all depends on what you do around and outside of my guidelines. You guys asked, so here it is! A book full of answers to all the questions I get on a daily basis!

So are you ready to do this with me? 30 DAYS! Commit to it, and I'm almost sure you're gonna want to keep going after that first month. 😊 The great news is, you can just repeat the same thing over and over again.

All you really need is 1-2 hours a day (more or less, depending on what your plan is each day), whenever it's convenient for you and whatever is possible according to your schedule. Should be doable, right? Cut out some TV time or some of that scrolling through the Internet, and boom, there's your couple of hours!

Tomorrow is your Day 1. And I say tomorrow for a reason. Because even though the saying is "Don't push to tomorrow, what you can do today," I have noticed that for me, sometimes starting tomorrow instead of today, can be a good thing! A clear head and rest is sometimes just what you need to start something new. And do not beat yourself up about starting something tomorrow. As long as procrastination isn't a routine of yours, starting tomorrow is absolutely fine *every now and then*. Hell, most things we consider bad for us are absolutely fine every now and then and are only bad if they become habits. Remember that.

Make it a habit to pick days where you just have to get up and do it NOW. It's called BALANCE, which is what my life, and this book, is all about!

So I'm going to guide you through each day, simply adding to your diet and fitness routine, and you'll also by doing little things you may not be used to doing.

Changing something in your (most likely) routined life will make a difference. Even if it seems insignificant to do something for just an hour, the fact is this: You don't have to make big changes to change. A little goes a long way when we are trying to better ourselves. What matters is that you're doing something new everyday, for the next 30 days! And that alone is GOALS.

Day 1

Get Out Of The House!

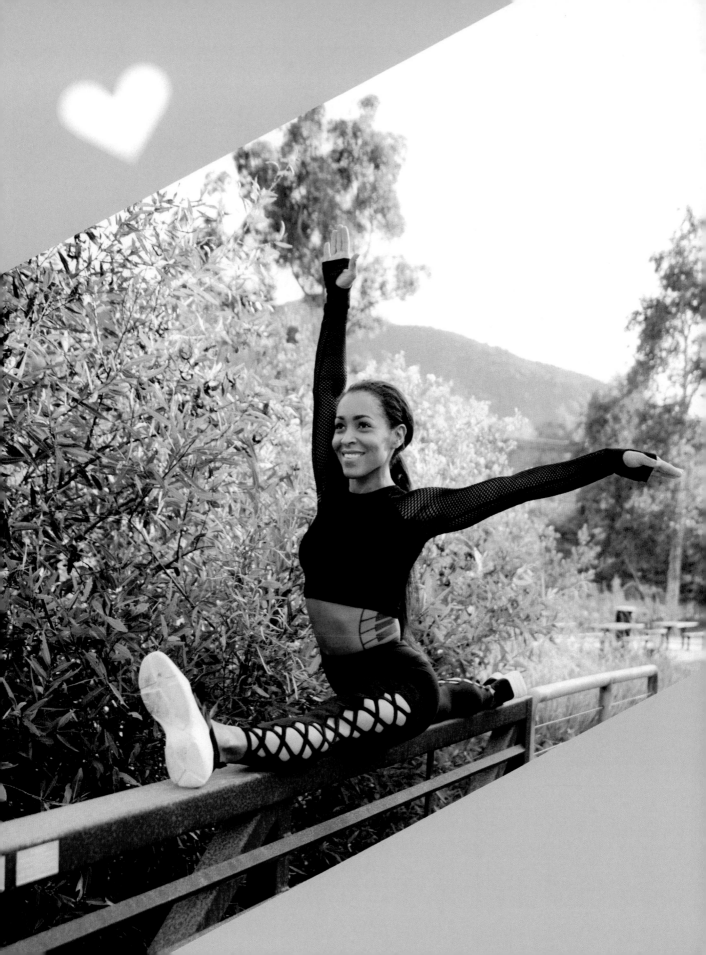

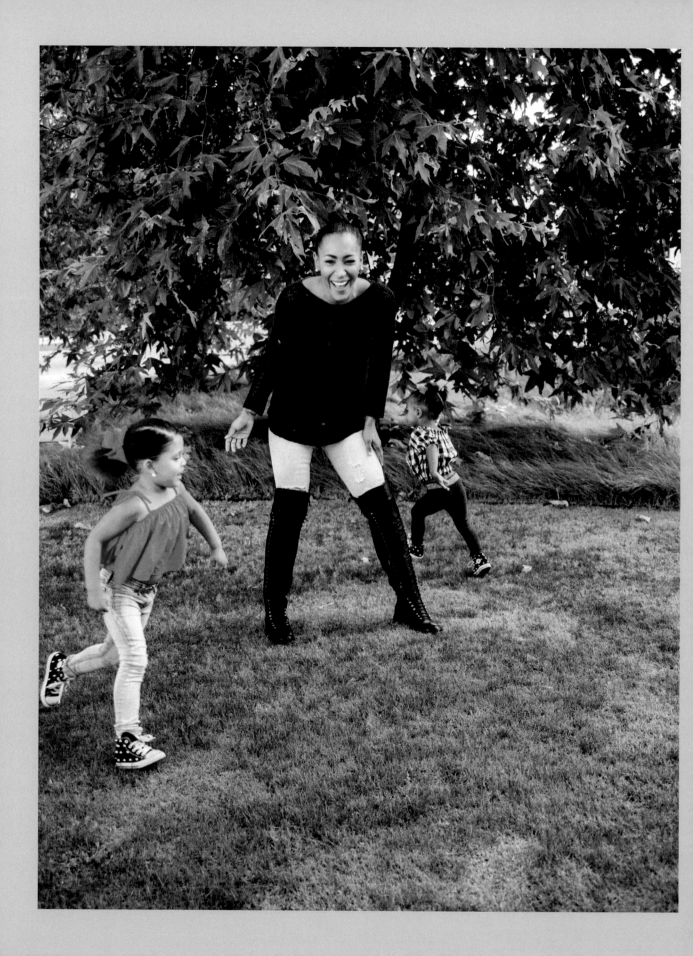

I am going to start by saying, I personally am an Outdoor Junkie! I don't know why, but ever since I was little I loved being outside. Most kids do. It's a natural thing for us to want to be outdoors every day, at least for a few hours. And that is why most of us get out. I started bringing both of my daughters outside within their first weeks of life and being that they were newborns, people thought I was crazy to be exposing them to germs, etc. However, I believed that nature, a little Vitamin D from the sun and fresh oxygen would do them just fine, as long as I kept them close to my body and not in direct exposure to anything that could harm them.

Being outside can initially change your mood. I know this might be a personal pet peeve of mine, but when I have to be in a room with artificial light during the day for a long time, I get anxiety. And I hardly ever get that. Being an artist, my sisters and I used to work in dark recording studios all the time, and I would always have to take breaks — like every 30 minutes — to step out and get some air. I know thousands of people work in of offices   every day without windows. And I do not envy them. It's something I could never do. Yes, many of us also live in places where there hardly is any good weather, so it doesn't always feel good to be outside. However, getting some air is something that is always of benefit for your well-being, even if you 'freeze your ass off' or get drenched.

Task : Today we are spending at least one hour outside. And this doesn't include your errands, going to work, going to an appointment or whatever else you have to do today. More than likely, you are headed out already, but whatever your schedule might be, even if you already have a long day outside planned, take an hour and just BE outdoors. It can be a place of your choice, with the people of your choice — your children, your significant other, yourself. It is completely up to you. No activity is necessary. You can just walk somewhere or sit somewhere and people-watch.

What you do with that one hour is your decision. What matters is that you are outdoors and that you don't spend the entire time in your phone. You may even want to put it away.

Be aware of your surroundings; look at the buildings, the trees, the cars, the sand. If you're lucky enough to be near a beach, that's even better. Just BE. Try no not think about your problems.

Make a conscious choice that for the next 30 days (and hopefully long after that) you will focus on what all the positive changes you make can bring into your life.

Yogurt Breakfast Bowl

FOOD OF THE DAY

A Great way to start any day! It's super easy to make, healthy and delicious! What more do we want? I used to not be much of a Yoghurt person, but after finding the perfect combinations in my favorite toppings, I love to make this bowl. Switching up the fruit each time makes it fun. You can literally use any fresh fruit you like. I never feel too full or bloated after having this. It always gives me just the right energy kick in the morning! Enjoy!

What you need
(for one bowl):

1 ½ cup of low-fat greek yogurt (Plain)

1 peach (substitute apple/pear/clementines)

half a cup of blueberries (or any other berries)

half a cup of almonds (substitute walnuts/vhazelnuts/cashews)

1 teaspoon coconut flakes

2 teaspoons honey

half a teaspoon cinnamon

Prep: 6 min, Cook: 0 min, Total Time: 6 min

Prepare:

1. Put the yogurt into the bowl

2. Wash and cut up the peach into small dices

3. Chop up almonds

4. Place all of the fruit and nuts into the bowl

5. Top it with the honey, cinnamon and coconut flakes

Stir, or eat as is. DONE

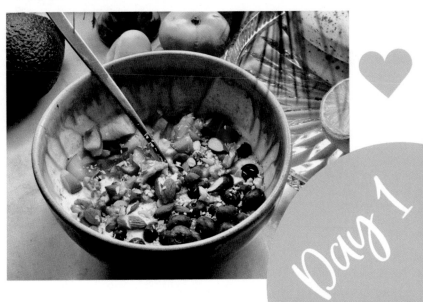

Day 1

Day 2

Wear Yourself Out!

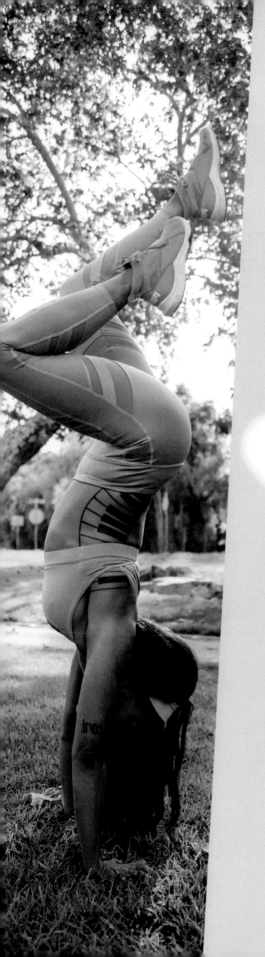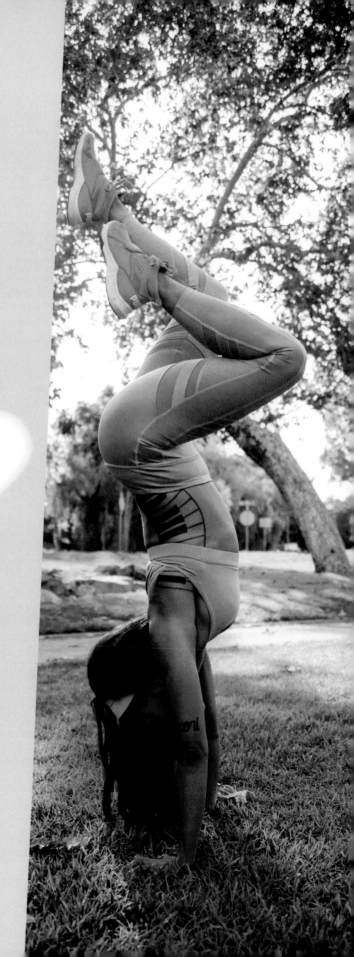

Hello, Beautiful. It's time to get to work! Today, the main thing is to exhaust yourself physically! Whatever time of day you decide to pick to follow this guide, get ready to put your workout attire on and bring your heart rate up!

One thing I've noticed over the years is that I'm more likely to work out if I'm already dressed accordingly. What also helps is getting myself a cute

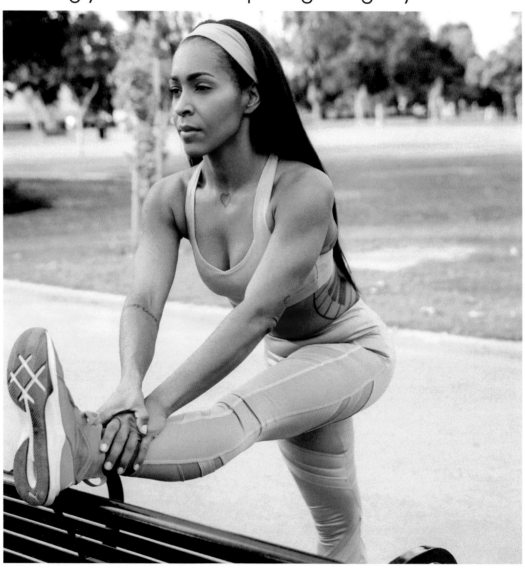

new, little fitness outfit which, yes, I know, requires a budget — so it's optional.

Anyway, Your Options Today are as Follows:

1. If you do have a gym membership and they offer classes, find a high intensity cardio and strength class such as HITT. You can also find classes like this at clubs like Barry's Bootcamp or Orange Theory Fitness.

2. Do at least 30 minutes on the treadmill, run (tempo 6/7/8 mph) for 2 minutes, then walk (tempo 3/4/5 mph) 2 minutes, then back to running and so on, and so on. After that, get yourself some 5-8 lb. weights and follow the FULL BODY routine on the next page.

> Do every exercise for 45 sec, then take 15 sec rest and move on to the next. Do at least 2 rounds, if you got it in you, 3 rounds!!

3. If you absolutely have no budget for a gym and/or no one to watch your kids, guess what? Your living room is about to —be your training ground! Go to YouTube and type in: "High Intensity workout," and you will see a bunch of workouts — mostly around 30 minutes — and you'll need nothing other than your body! You will be doing this twice today, morning and night or back-to-back. It's your choice. What matters is that for one hour you're working hard today - so hard that you won't want to do anything else! I promise this is just one of the few days we will go HAM!

Day 2

Deadlift & Row

Standing position, feet hips width apart with a slight bend in the knees and holding the dumbbells, bend your upper body forward with a straight back while pushing the butt backwards. dumbbells close to the floor, come half way up so your back is paralell to the floor, hold and row both arms keeping the ellblows close to the body. Straighten arms, and with a flat back stand back up straight. repeat.

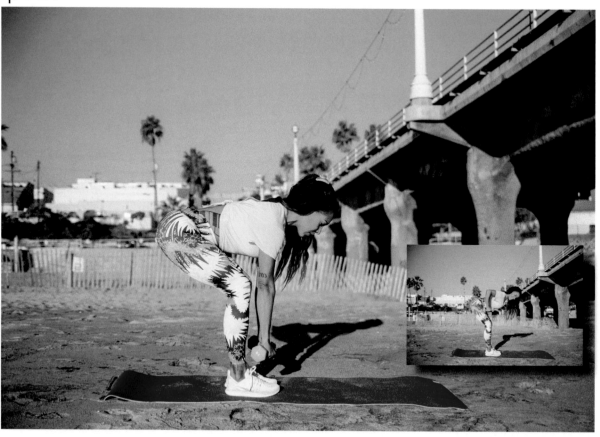

Russian Twist ♥

Sit down on the floor, lean back 45 degrees and lift up your feet off of the floor using your abdominal muscles. Twist your upper body left and right holding your dumb-bells. Modify by using only one dumbell in front of your chest.

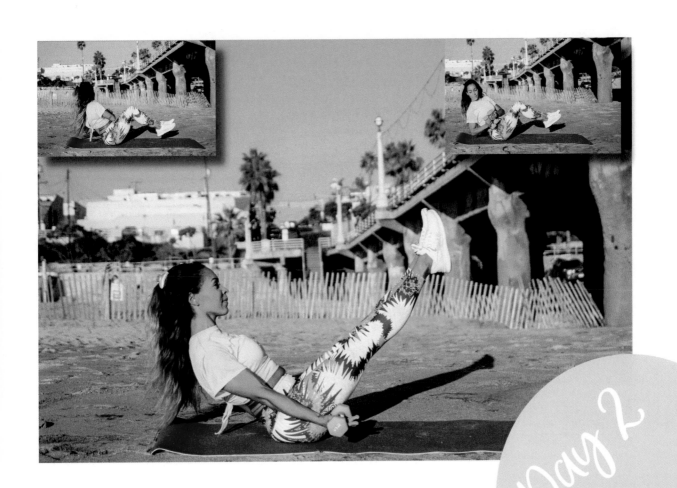

Day 2

Reverse Fly

Standing position, dumbbells in hand. Bend forward half way with a slight bend in the knees. Open up your arms to the side wide squeezing your shoulder blades together. Slowly and controlled bring them back down to meet eachother

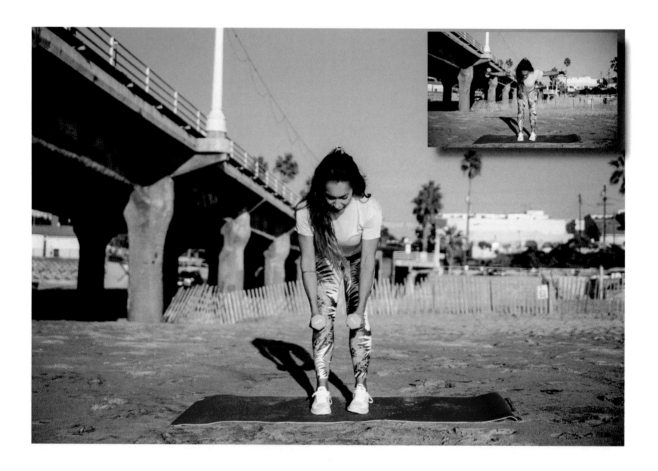

Forward & Reverse Lunge

Standing position, lunge forward with the right leg, left knee should almost be touching the floor, upper body is straight. Bring the right foot back to meet the left, then lunge back with the same leg. After 45 sec, switch legs.

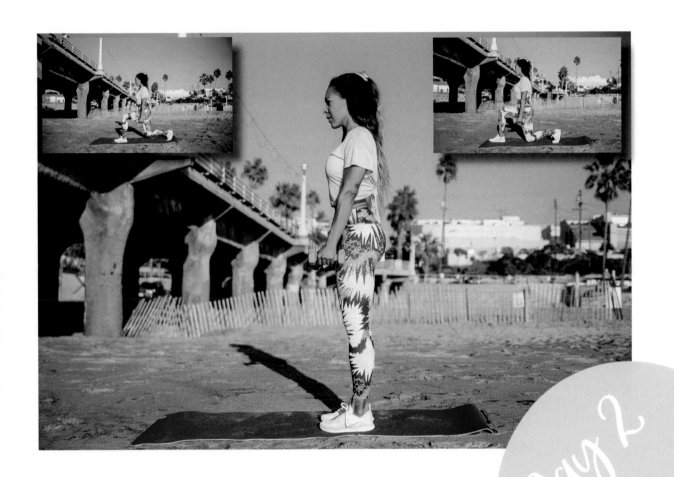

Day 2

Plank Row

Plank position, wrists directly under your shoulders, place your hands onto the dumbbells and row left and right while keeping the core engaged the entire time.

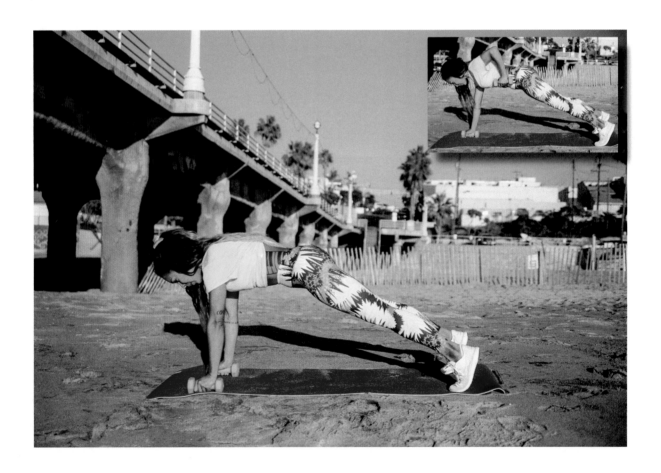

High Plank-Toe Touch

Start in HIGH plank position, wrists directly under your shoulders, keep your hips low (straight body!), engage your core to move your hips up with straight legs while pushing the chest towards feet. Touch opposite hand to opposit ankle alternating back and forth to the high plank position. Make sure you do not bend your knees here.

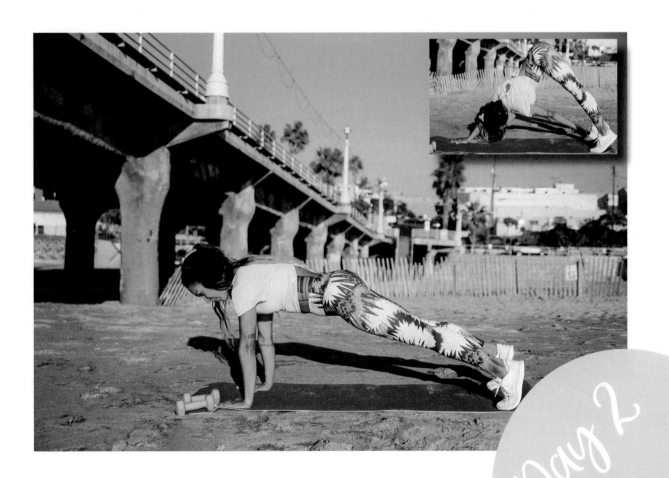

Day 2

Jump Squat

Start in standing position. Dumbbells in hand but keep your arms down and close to the body. jump up as high as you can and land in squat, jump up right away from squat and land back in squat! When you jump, push off your heels!

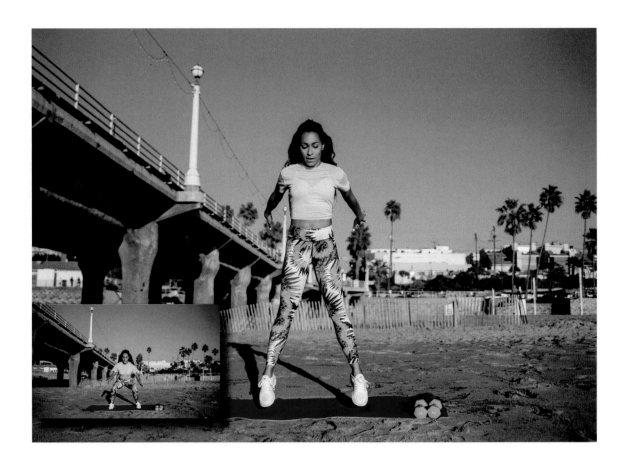

Double Squat ♥

Stand up straight, place your feet a little wider than your hips and always keep your weight mostly on the heels. toes pointing forward, squat down, pulse up half way, then back down and come all the way up back to standing. Jump your feet together and repeat the same move this time with the feet side by side. Then go back to opening the feet and so on. Hold your dumbbells in fron of your chest or on your shoulders. Make sure when you squat you don't bring your knees forward!! But your hips back!! Also keep the chest up

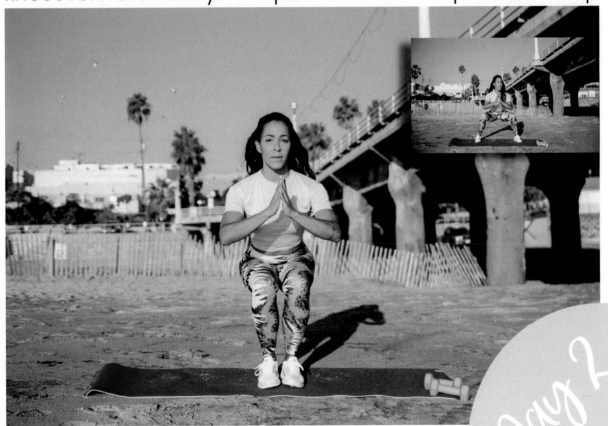

Day 2

30

Push-Up Walk Up

Start in push up position, bend your elbows , then move your chest towards the ground while keeping the ellbows close to the body, push up and walk your hands back to your ankles. Walk them back out to push up position. repeat. (modify by going on to your knees if a regular push up is too hard for you).

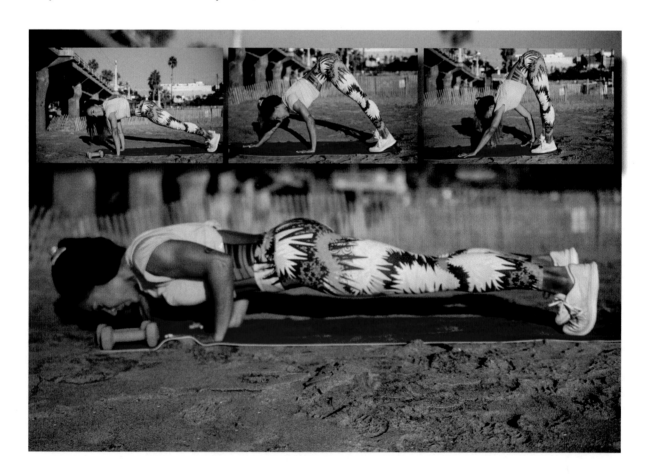

If your kids are around while you workout, make them understand that this is something very important to you and that working out is what mommy needs right now. Promise them a surprise for later if they be good kids and let you do what you're doing for 30 min. Also, over time they will understand that this is just what happens in your household - just like you doing your makeup or watching a show you like. The more they get used to it, the more they will accept it, give you your time and "behave" during your workout. Just keep at it! You won't regret it.

Day 2

Food Of The Day

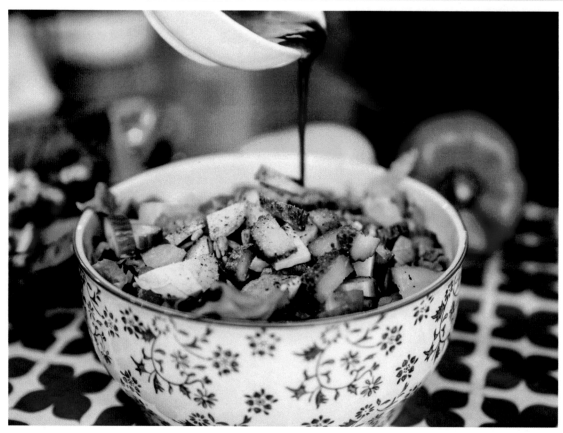

Hello, Salad! This should definitely be a go-to meal for you! I make so many different salads (probably could have a whole book of just salads), but the truth is, most of the salads I make are the same, just with add-ons or a substituted green! When you make salad all the time you   wanna test out different flavors in it. I may use olives one day and dried cranberries the next. I may use feta cheese today and shredded cheddar tomorrow; tuna on Monday and add grilled chicken on Tuesday! Or, I'll add some bacon and a hard boiled egg, and boom, I've made me a Cobb salad. It really is so simple. My salads all have the same Dressing: MY HOUSE DRESSING that everyone has been asking me about for months now. My dressing goes with all of them! This recipe is the "basic" recipe with the ingredients I pretty much always use! No meat, no extras just plain , Simple salad! Enjoy!

Simple Salad & Homemade Dressing

Prep:10 min, Cook:0 min, Total Time:10min

What You need (for 2 servings):

1 head of romaine lettuce

1 big tomato or 4-5 grape tomatoes

2 persian cucumbers

2 dill pickles

½ red, yellow or orange pepper

½ avocado

2 tablespoons of sunflower seeds

salt and pepper

For the dressing:

⅓ cup of Olive Oil

¼ cup of balsamic vinegar

1 teaspoon honey

1 teaspoon yellow mustard

1 teaspoon low-fat greek yoghurt

salt, pepper and garlic powder for seasoning

Prepare.

Wash the lettuce and cut off the bottom end, then cut it up and place into bowl. Wash and cut up all of the other raw ingredients into small pieces and mix into bowl.

The Dressing:

In a separate small bowl, combine all the ingredients and stir well. Pour over salad and mix the entire contents, serve right away.

Day 2

Day 3

Have fun with it!

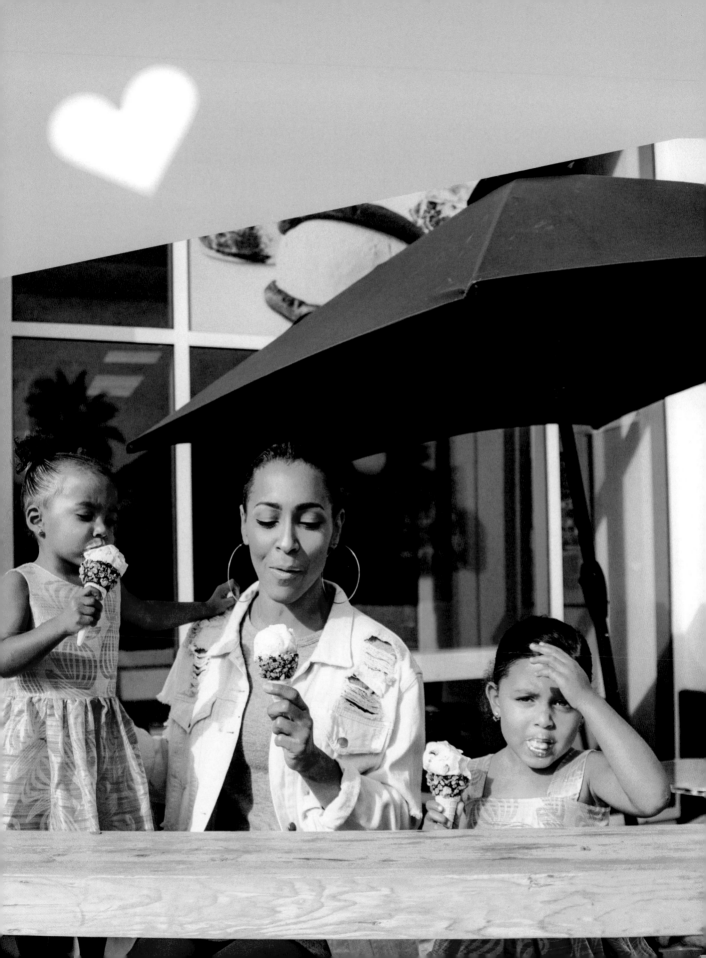

Although today we are not focused on working out, I encourage you to still get some cardio in.That's what I would do! A 20-30 minute light jog is good enough and will make a difference in your overall experience with this challenge . . . I promise. So if possible, do that to begin the day!

MOMMY TIP!

If you have no way to get to a treadmill or jog outside because you're with your kids all day, get yourself a rope and jump!!! If you have toddlers, like me, they love seeing mommy jump, it's one of their favorite things to do, and i'm sure they aren't used to seeing you jump like a kid. 😉

How?

If jumping is all I do for my cardio I normally like to start at:

50 jumps, take a minute.

60 jumps, take another minute.

70 jumps

80 jumps

90 jumps

100 jumps (finally)

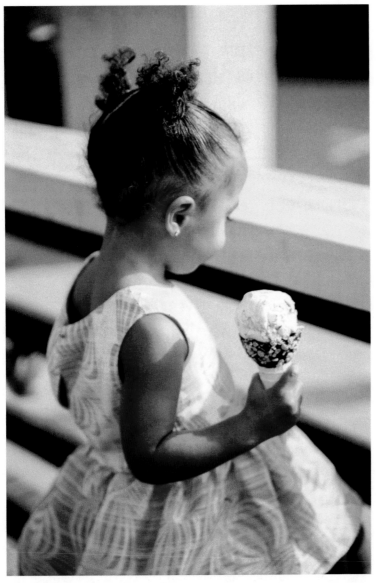

Of course if you normally never, *ever* jump, don't start at 50, like me. You can start at 30 or even 20, but make sure you increase every time you start a new set. Breaks can be longer once you go up in numbers, but you have to finish! And push yourself! Don't be lazy. 😉

Day 3

Another tip: If you have kids running around, like I do, put on music that they enjoy and make it a dance party while you jump rope. Have FUN with it, even if you don't feel like it, *act as* if it's fun for you. It helps . . . and time will fly by. You will be amazed and feel like you accomplished a goal afterwards!! Now, if you have a busy day ahead of you with lots of running around to do, you are excused from the next task of the day. But if you don't work a 9-5 job and are a full-time mom, like me, plan an activity with the kids! It doesn't have to cost a dollar. You can go to the park with them and play hide and seek! Don't sit on the bench looking in your phone! If you have errands to run, take the kids with you.

I encourage you, even if you have someone who can watch them at home while you run your errands, take them with you instead! Yes, it may be easier not to, but trust me when I say, it's BET-TER when you do — for you and the kids. It's more work for you, but the key thing here is that we want more physical activity! I break into a sweat getting my kids into their car-seats and the stroller into the trunk almost everyday, which I'm not even phased about anymore. I am certain that because I am constantly being active by doing things like this, I have been more in shape than before my kids were born. And the best part is the kids are happier when they get to go out with mommy! They may say they like to stay home, but most likely they will just watch

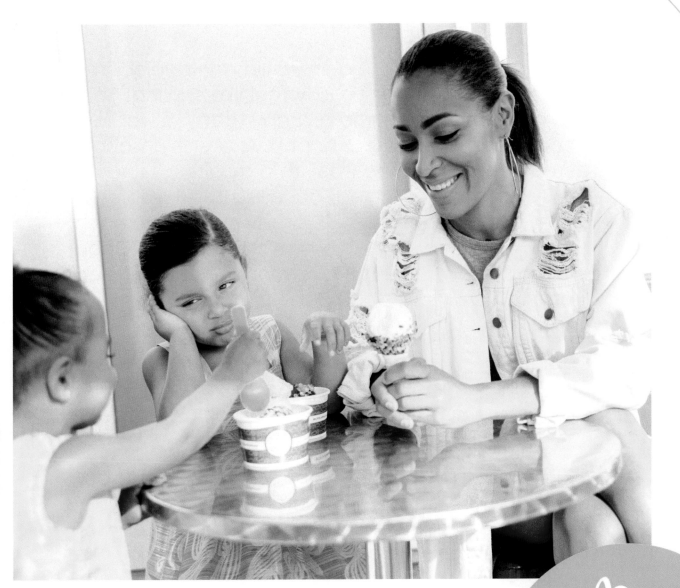

Day 3

TV or play video games — and there is enough time to do that later!! So, pack up your babies and GO - with a smile on your face!

I've learned to put a smile on my face, for my kids, even when I don't really feel like smiling! So if you happen to be a little grumpy today or not in a good mood, try ACTING happy. And stay in character! I actually came up with a tradition. (and it's the most beautiful thing, because the happiness on my daughters' faces just drops over to me each morning.) I open the blinds and start singing "Good Morning, Good Morning, Good Morning to you, Good Morning, how you doing? Cock-a-doodle-doo!!"

Every single morning, my kids wake up to me singing. I just know they will forever remember these times and having memories like this equals HAPPI-NESS. And their happiness is My Happiness!

There is a quote by someone unknown I recently came across which reads, "We smile because we are happy, but we also become happy because we smile". Unless you're a completely depressed person (which hopefully isn't you) smiling works! And you learn it how? Like everything you want to learn - by doing it!

Brown Rice with Curry sauce & Broccoli

FOOD OF THE DAY

Prep:0min, Cook:20min, Total Time:20min

Prepare:

1. In a pot, place the rice and add 4 cups of water

2. Bring to a boil and immediately lower the heat to LOW.

3. Cover the pot with a lid and let it simmer for 15-20min until water has resolved. Stir occasionally.

4. In a separate pot, heat the butter til it's melted and whisk in the flour

5. immediately add the milk and keep whisking

6. Add Broth and all seasonings while stiring on medium heat

7. Cut up Broccoli florets if they're too big, otherwise just add them as is and keep on medium heat for another 5-7 min

8. When done, sprinkle with parsley! DONE

9. Serve combined in medium size bowls. YUM!

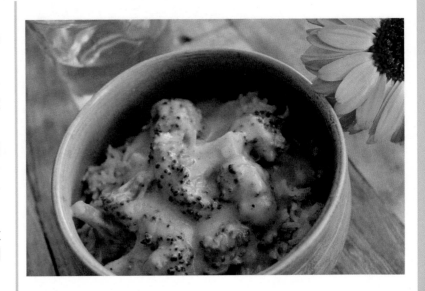

2 cups of brown rice

5oz fresh broccoli florets

2 cups of milk

2 tablespoons butter (substitute coconut oil for healthier option)

2 tablespoons flour

1 tablespoon broth (any kind)

salt and pepper

curry powdwer

fresh or frozen Parsley

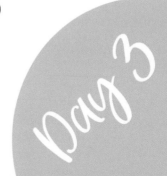

Day 3

Day 4

Stillness

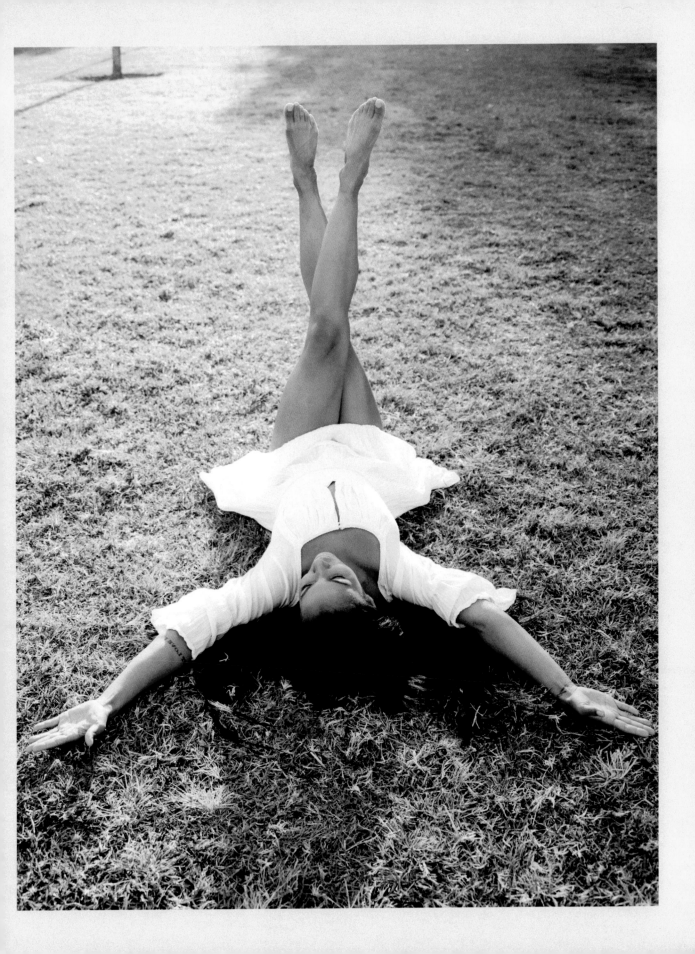

Be still...

Learning how to relax your mind and body is just as important to our overall wellness as the moving! I learned that when I started Yoga.

We are not practicing Asana (Yoga poses) today, unless you already know what you're doing and want to do the poses. If that's the case, go ahead! However, today is all about relaxation.

You may have a hectic day ahead of you, but relaxing (especially your mind), doesn't necessarily mean you have to do nothing. Go about your day! Go to work. Go do what you have to do, even go hit the gym, if you feel like it! But here are a few things that represent stillness to me. Things that I do when I need to release stress:

Day 4

Pause

Be especially mindful about taking "a breather" here and there today. "Take a moment". Put your phone down for five minutes and look at the sky while you think about your biggest dreams. You can do this multiple times throughout the day. Yes, there is ALWAYS something to do, especially for us moms, but it is okay to *sometimes* occupy your kids with a movie so that you can 'take a moment'.

Important Tip: Take a break from scrolling through social media, even if it's just for a few hours.

Day 4

In preparation for tomorrow's first Yogi Day, whenever time permits today (even if you have to wait until your kids have gone to bed) find a quiet place, sit upright and take long deep breaths with your eyes and mouth closed. Find focus in this breath which is exactly what we will be using in YOGA...UJJAYI breath, which is a steady breath you control by simply closing your mouth and being more attentive to it than you are when you breathe normally. This is great to do prior to the yoga exercise I have for us tomorrow! Try not to have your mind wander and try not to think about all you've got to do and/or your problems. In other words, exhale the BS, and just BE. You know how amazing it can be to just breathe? I never realized how amazing it feels until I focused all my energy on my breathing and let go of everything for a few minutes

Breathe

Day 4

Be Patient

Make today the "First Day of Different" when it comes to reacting.

If your kids are getting on your nerves, don't yell. If your boss is being annoying, brush it off and keep the day going. If your boyfriend or husband is being a pain in your ass, smile and go. Yes, it takes everything in me to sometimes to keep calm when my girls are not listening or making a huge mess in the house, but today we are not raising our voice, no matter what. Think you can't do it? Well how about giving it a try!

I have found myself getting aggravated about little things numerous times, and in the end it didn't change a thing. But maybe gave me a few grey hairs and a headache.

Day 4

This goes together with Tip #2. At any given moment today, when you want to say something, stop and think about whether or not it is necessary to say! A good quote to follow is, "Don't speak unless you can improve the silence." This is our motto today: Challenge yourself, and maybe one day you can live your life knowing that everything that comes out of your mouth will be valuable and worth saying!

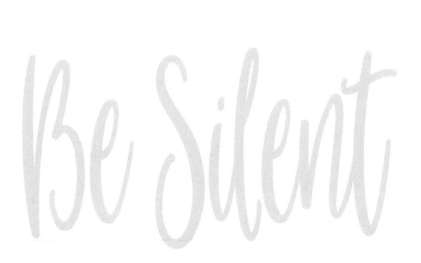

Be Silent

Day 4

TOMATO SOUP
(Blender required)

Most kids (and adults) will love this dish! My nephews in Germany would basically eat this for breakfast lunch and dinner, and they are also the ones who have gotten my daughters hooked! It's great for dipping as well with some fresh, whole grain baguette or simply toast! Low calorie but filling and that is always a winner!!

What you need:-
3-4 tablespoons olive oil
1 large onion
2 medium sized carrots
1 red pepper
2 large cans of tomatoes (whole)

300ml vegetable broth
fresh basil
salt and pepper
dash of chili powder
2 tablespoons sugar (or a sugar substitute)
cream to taste (or vegan cream)

Prepare:

1.Add chopped onion, pepper and carrots - close lid - reduce heat to med.

2.Let simmer for 2-3 mins while stiring sometimes.

3.Add canned tomatoes and broth.

4.Add spices and sweetener.

5.Simmer on medium/low with covered lid for about 10-15 mins (stirring occasionally).

6.Add chopped (or frozen) basil and cream (or cream replacement) and turn off heat. Let cool down a bit and then.

7.Blend until even, (Add more water or broth if too thick).

Enjoy

Day 4

Day 5

Yogi Day

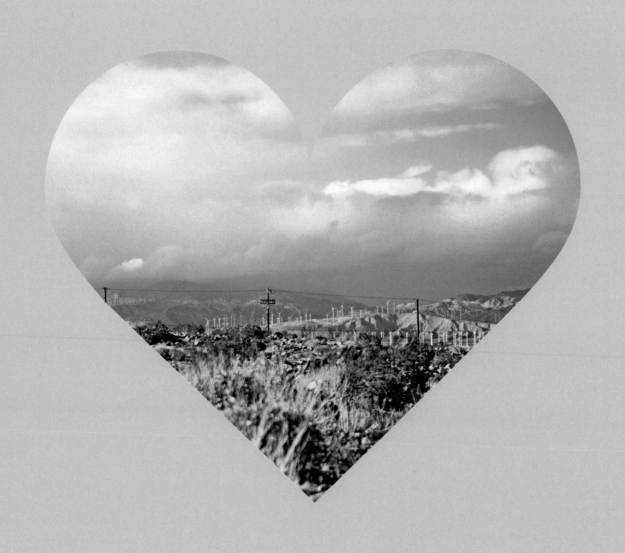

Ever since I started posting and sharing my yoga poses and exercises, I've been getting e-mails and messages from women asking me how I got started! Well, honestly, I just took a yoga class one day. I wanted to explore something different when it came to my workout regimen. I've always been about my fitness, but in my early 20s all I would ever do is run, and then do some sit-ups, push-ups and those type of exercises. I never knew or thought that yoga could interest me, even though I was aware that I had always been pretty flexible. I just never thought that I could be challenged in something like yoga. And challenge was what I was into.

However, that completely changed after my first class. A big reason may be that my first yoga class ever was a Bikram Yoga class, which is a very intense 90 minute yoga class in a room that has a temperature of around 90 degrees. It included 26 poses that have a set order, then repeated in the exact same way each class. Most people who try it, struggle to even stay in the hot room for the entire 90 minutes. But with me being super competitive (not with others, but with myself), I loved the fact that it was hard . . . super hard!! It was much different from what I had expected. I also was amazed at how cleansed and refreshed I felt after class. I felt like a new person. I literally felt like a Superhero! It got to a point where I would take Bikram 4-5 days a week. And I remember ditching all of my running and other forms of work-outs I had done before. The only thing I wanted and the only thing my body was craving was Bikram Yoga. Those were the days! I was in amazing shape! However, over the years, and especially after becoming a mom, I have been interested in exploring other styles of yoga! There are so many! And I am still learning about a lot of them! I do feel that a basic Vinyasa flow is a great way to start learning poses and breathing and just to get Into It. If you're a complete beginner I have come up with a flow that should be simple enough to follow by pictures and description.

Now, I am not a certified yoga instructor and I do encourage you to find a nice yoga studio and take a class, or multiple classes if you like it (just for the experience) because doing yoga in a group can be such an amazing and different experience. What I am showing you in this book is what I do, when I practice alone (or with my kids running around, which does require extra focus and the ability to zone out while still being attentive). Whew!! Not easy, I tell ya. But POSSIBLE! And no worries, you are learning real poses that I learned from certified teachers and self-study. But yoga isn't about doing things right, it's about doing things that are right for you and your body. It's about becoming more aware of your body. There is no such thing as the perfect yogi because, guess what? You are perfect the way you are now and perfectly fine to do yoga, even if you cannot touch the ground with your fingers and with your legs straight! Even if you weigh more than you should, yoga is for EVERYONE. That is the first thing you need to know!

You do what you can and no one is judging you! At least not us yogis!

Yoga Sequence (FLOW)
What you need: A mat & 30 minutes.

Day 5

60

1. Cat/Cow

Start on all fours, with hands and knees, and the top of your feet on the mat. Make sure your shoulders are positioned directly above your wrists and your hips above your knees. INHALE up into cow by curving your spine down and looking up at the sky. When your lungs are full, exhale slowly while reversing into cat by pulling in your belly, tilt your pelvis and bringing your chin to your chest. Hold it, then INHALE back into cow. Do this about ten times and take your time. Try to take super slow, deep breaths and move in sync with them.

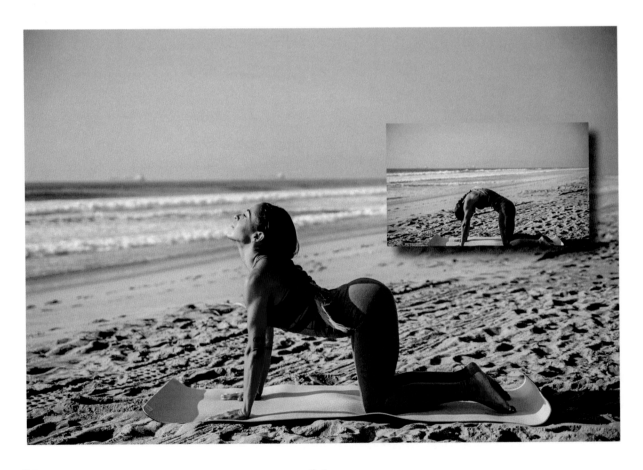

2. Downdog

From All fours and a nutural spine, tuck under your toes and press up into Downward Facing Dog. Place your feet hip-width apart onto the mat and straighten your legs (your heels don't have to touch the mat, but encourage them to do so). Move your chest down to the floor while exhaling, then stay there and continue to breathe. Bend one knee at a time and walk it out for a few breath cycles. Move your hips around, but keep anchored on your mat through your hands and feet! We are warming up the hips, the shoulders and wrists while getting a good stretch in the back of our legs.

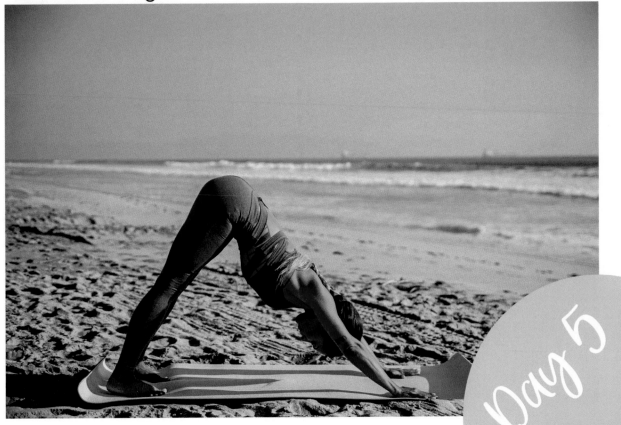

Day 5

3. Plank

From Downdog, straighten yourself out into a Plank. Shoulders should be exactly above the wrists with a protracted back, (shoulder blades apart and away from eachother). You are on your toes and your heels press towards the back. Your head is straight (not up or down) and you're looking right in-between your hands. Go back and forth between Plank and Downdog a few times while breathing slow before moving on to the next pose.

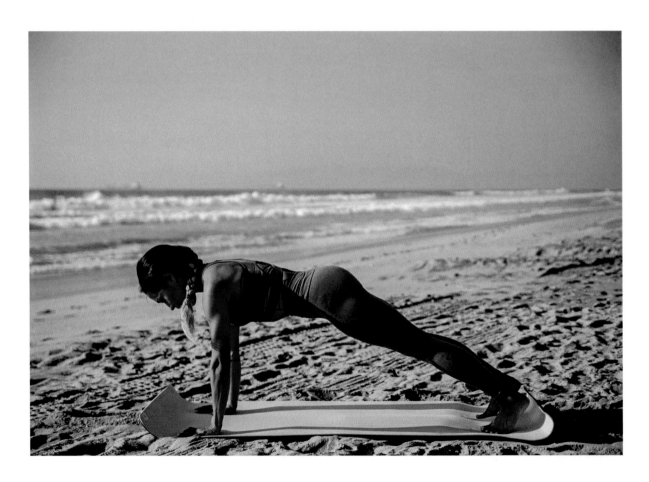

4. Chaturanga

From Plank, shift forward 'til your shoulders are above your fingertips and lower down by bending your elbows like you're about to do a push-up. Hold the elbows in close to the sides of your body (important) stop and hold a few inches off the ground. Inhale and move into cobra (see next posture).

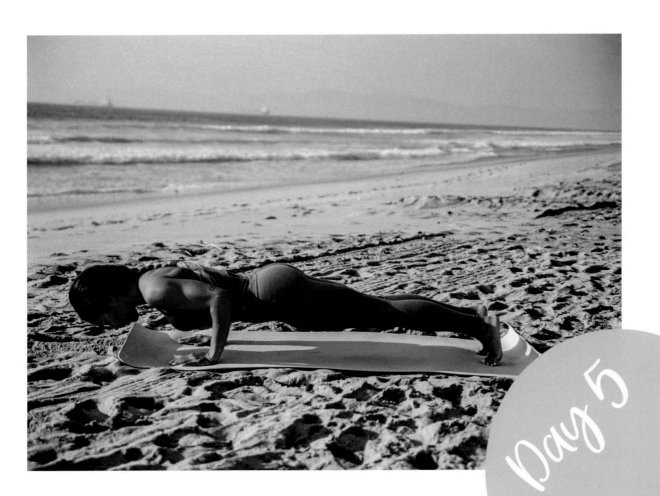

Day 5

5. Cobra

Flip your toes and touch your belly onto the mat, in other words come all the way down onto the mat and immediately push your upper body back up by using your back and arm strength. Inhale. Keep your elbows in! And look up to the sky. Do not straighten your arms out all the way keep a slight bend in them and try to really focus on using back strength to 70 percent and 30 percent arm strength. From here, push back into a Downdog and repeat Plank, Chaturanga and Cobra about 3-5 times. Remember, move slow! Breathe deep!

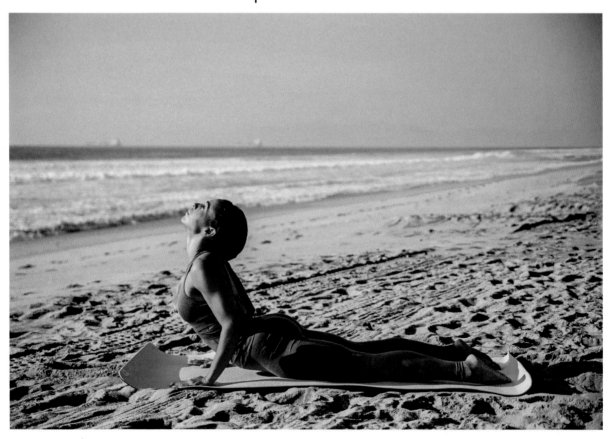

6. One Legged Dog Knee To Chest

After a few cycles, from Downdog, lift your right leg up to the sky and hold it. On an exhale, come forward to a Plank without setting the right foot down. Bend your knee towards the chest and try touching your forehead. Push back up into One Legged Dog. Repeat 5 times.

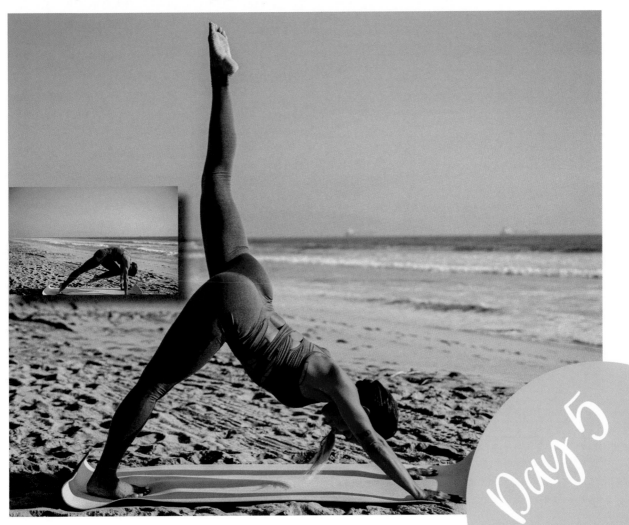

Day 5

66

7. Warrior 1 To Extended Warrior 1

After the 5th cycle, place your right foot in-between your hands, and place your left foot down flat on the mat in a 45-degree angle. Slowly rise up with a straight back and your arms above your head with palms facing each other. Keep your shoulders down! Activate your glutes on the left side so that the weight is equally distributed be- tween both legs. Your right knee is bent exactly above the ankle. BREATHE! Hold for about 10 seconds then keep your lower body (hips down), and only move your upper body forward 45 degrees until you achieve a straight line from left heel to fingertips! Hold, again, while breathing.

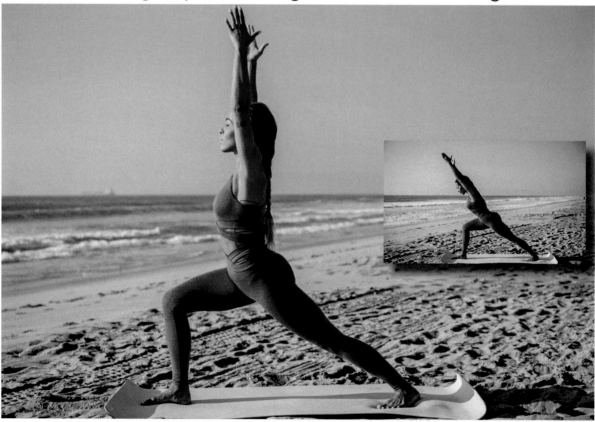

8. Warrior 2

From Extended Warrior, turn your chest sideways and extend your arms out parallel to the floor with the palms facing down. Legs will stay in the same position, but move your hips to the same side as your chest. Make sure that your right knee is exactly over your ankle and not bowing out to the left or right. Turn your head back to the front, looking past your right hand. Breathe! Stay in this position for about 5 breath cycles.

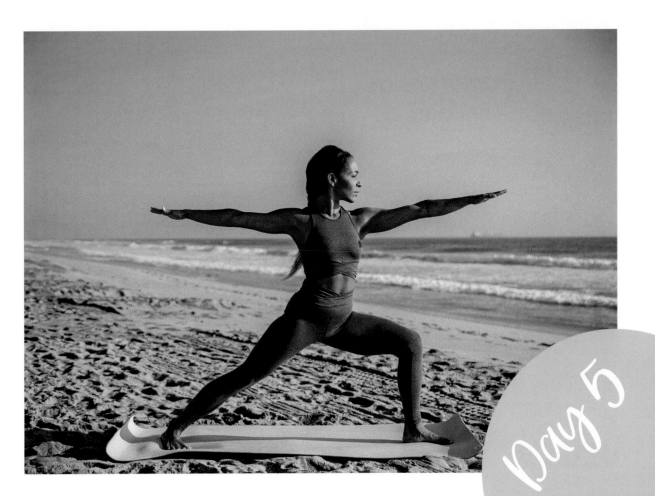

Day 5

9. Reverse Warrior 2

On an exhale, drop your back hand down to the back thigh while keeping the arm straight. Simultaneously lift the opposite arm straight up towards the sky. The lifted arms bicep should be right by your ear and your gaze is up past your hand. Keep the hips low as you lengthen up your entire spine (try to not sink in too much into the back side but rather think UP and lengthen. Hold and breathe for about 10 breaths. Then go back to Warrior 2.

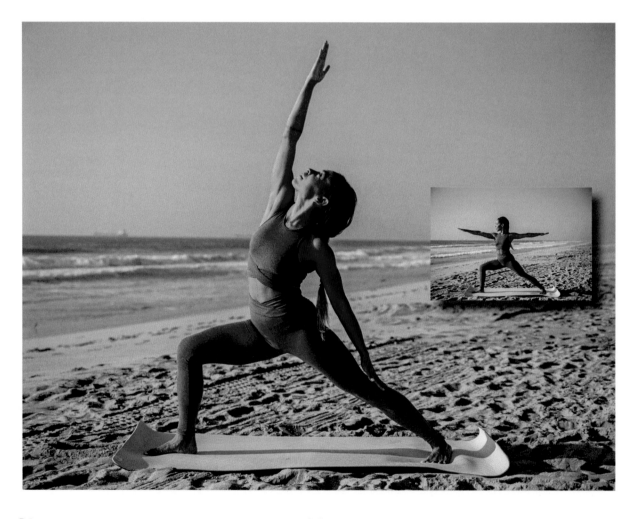

10. Bikram Triangle To Triangle

From Warrior 2, stretch your front arm down to your front toes aligning the elbow exactly at your knee, no higher, no lower. Lift the back arm up into the sky and twist at the waist. Open up your chest without curving your spine. Keep a straight line from your back heel to your underarm. Be stable in your lower body, still distributing weight equally. Look up to the sky and take deep breaths in and out your nose.

Then slowly straighten your bent knee and let your bottom wrist hover at the shin. Keep everything else the same. You should be feeling a major twist. If you feel like your upper body is bending forward ensure that its in a straight line with the rest of your body.

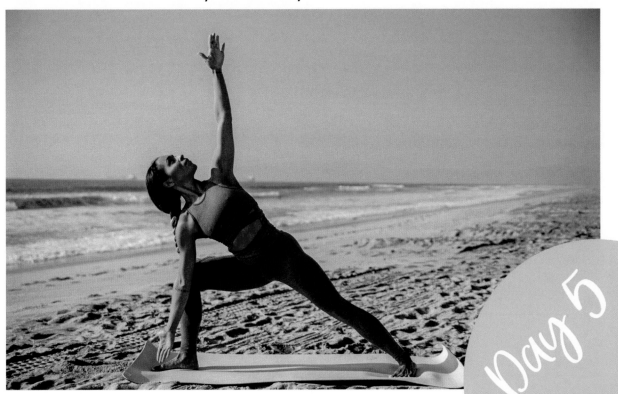

Day 5

70

11. Half Moon

From Triangle, lift off the back leg parallel to the floor as you place the bottom fingertips on the floor. You can bend the standing leg, but work on straightening it once you're in posture. Stretch the top arm into a straight line up into the sky and open your chest into the same direction you're facing, then look up towards the top hand, stay in position and breathe (5 breaths)! Then slowly bend the standing leg and place the top foot back down, landing in triangle (previous pose).

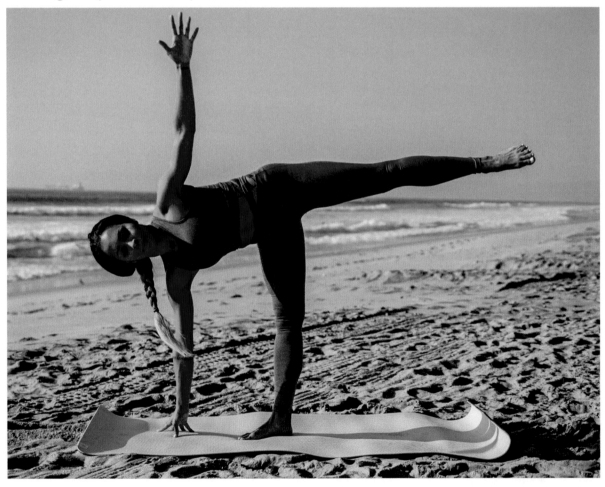

12. One Legged Plank

From Triangle, bend the front leg, and frame your foot with both of your hands on the floor into a low lunge. Put the weight into your hands and bring the front leg back, but don't put it down! Instead, keep it up in the air straight (with no bent knee). Muscles should contract with a pointed foot while the rest of your body is in the Plan position. Hold. Breathe (about 3 breaths).

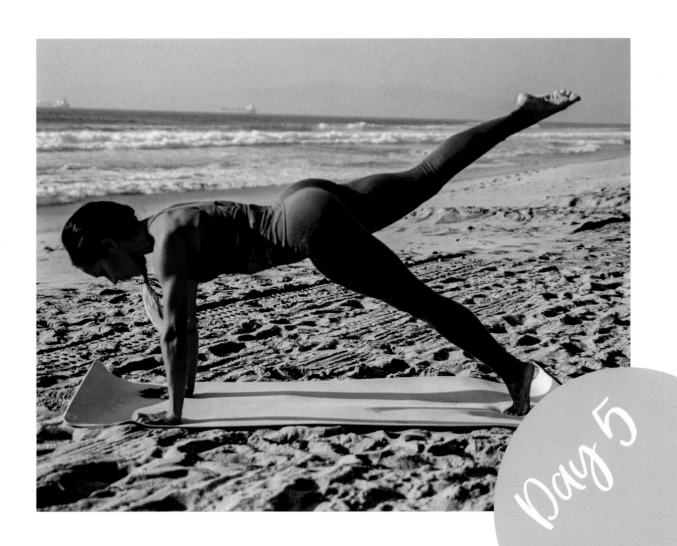

13. Upward Facing Dog

From One-Legged Plank, move through Chaturanga to Up Dog. You get to this posture by pressing your palms on the floor and lifting your upper body. Drag the hips slightly forward and un-curl your toes so that the top of your feet are flat on the floor. Inhale as you go higher, open your chest and gaze into the sky. Keep your legs active and straight. Try to lift your knees off the floor while keeping everything else the same.

Switch side

From Up Dog move back into a Down Dog and go back to the beginning of this sequence, starting point 6. But this time, do the opposite side!

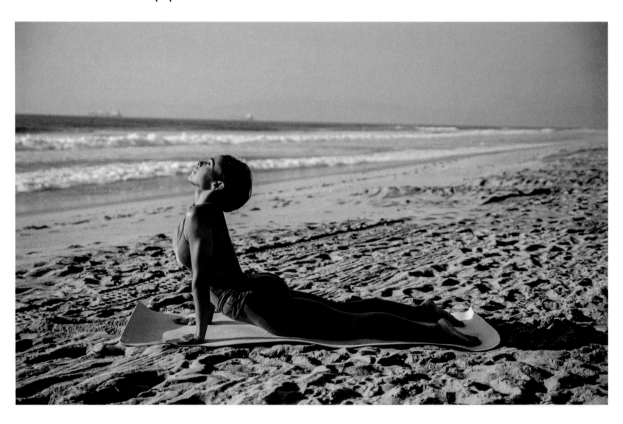

14. Side Plank

From down dog now, uncurl into plank then shift your weight into the right hand. Roll to the outside of your right foot and place your left foot on top of it (paralell). Lift up the left hand towards the sky. Try to keep your body in a straight line from toes to head.

Slowly slide the top foot up towards the calf and eventually the inner side of the knee without letting your top knee come forward, but rather point it up towards the sky. Stay here. Breathe slowly.

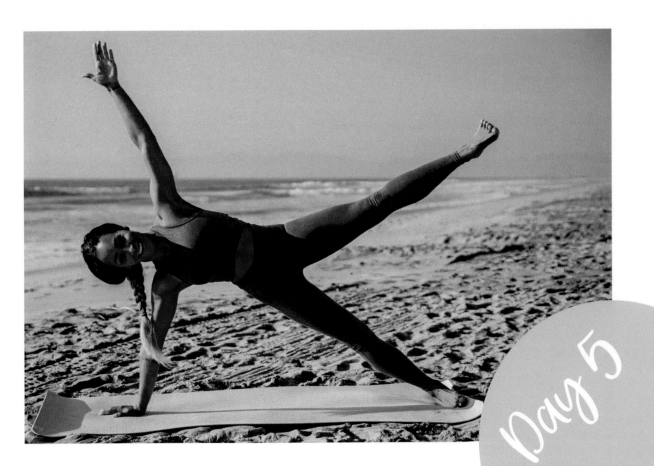

Day 5

15. Wild Thing

From side plank, release the ball of the foot onto the ground behind you, it should rest close underneath the hip. Keep the left leg extended. Make sure your legs are hip width apart as you reach the top hand overhead.

Lift your pelvis higher and let your head and neck fall back as far as they go. Relax into it. Open the chest. Take 5 breaths here. And exit by rotating back and turning the gaze back down to the floor, land in plank position.

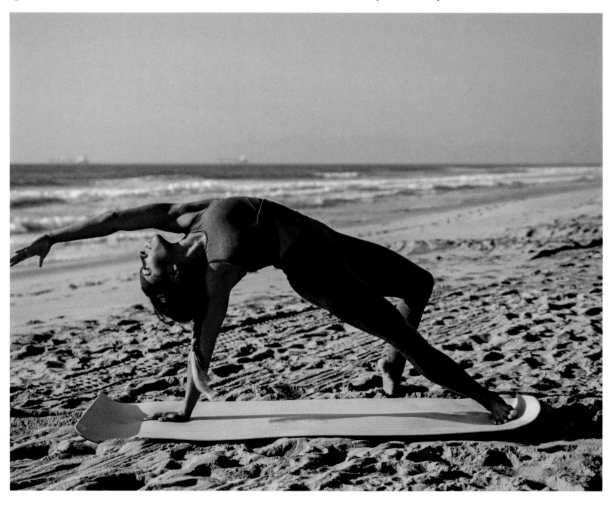

16. Puppy Pose

From Plank, put your knees on the mat. Place the top of your feet on the mat as well, and extend your hands a bit more forward on the mat. Lower your chest towards the ground while continuously stretching and activating your arms straight in front of you. Keep your hips above your knees and place your forehead on the mat. Breathe and feel your spine lengthening.

Switch sides

Slowly come back to a table top, curl your toes under and straighten your legs out to land in Plank. Repeat steps 14 and 15 on the left side, then get back into Puppy Pose, to Table Top, to Plank.

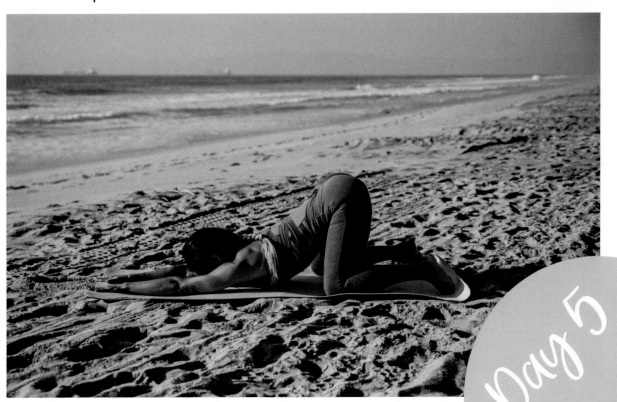

Day 5

17. Forward Fold

From Plank, walk yourself forward on your hands (you can have your knees bent). Try to touch the floor, but do not round your back. Keep your knees bent, and if you feel your back rounding, look towards the ground, then let your head hang heavy and walk it out for a few breaths. Rock side-to-side. Shake your head in yes and no gestures. Move your knees and head around while keeping the feet planted on the ground. Relax into it.

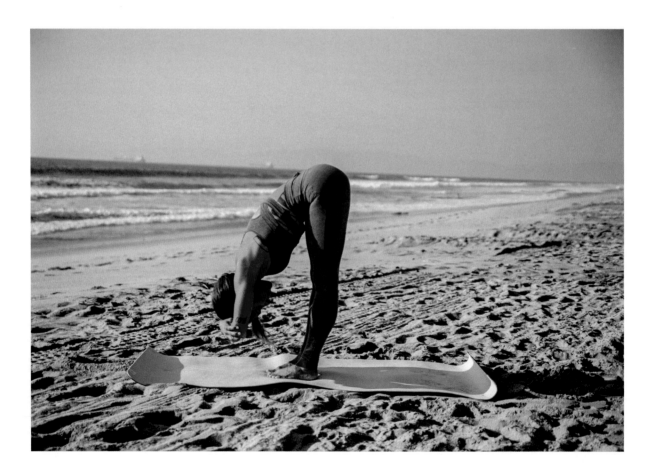

18. Chair Pose

From forward fold, bend your legs so that your chest touches your thighs with your hands still on the ground. Keep gazing to the floor as you bend the knees more until they are parallel to the floor. Now, lift your arms and chest forward and away from your thighs and distribute all your bodyweight on your heels. Sit back as if you are sitting in a chair while opening your chest. Extend your arms up to-wards the sky. Tilt your pelvis forward a bit until you feel your thighs working super hard. Breathe evenly and slowly through your nose 5-10 breaths.

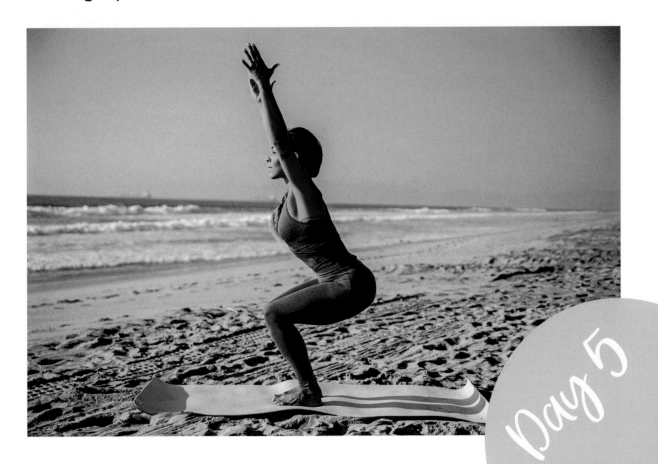

Day 5

19. Revolved Side Angle Prayer

From chair. Bring your hands into prayer by the heart. Twist at the waist as you keep your lower body strong (weight still in the heels). Place your right elbow onto the left knee keeping the length in your spine. Do not round. From here stretch your right foot all the way back behind you into a lunge position, take about 5 breaths here.

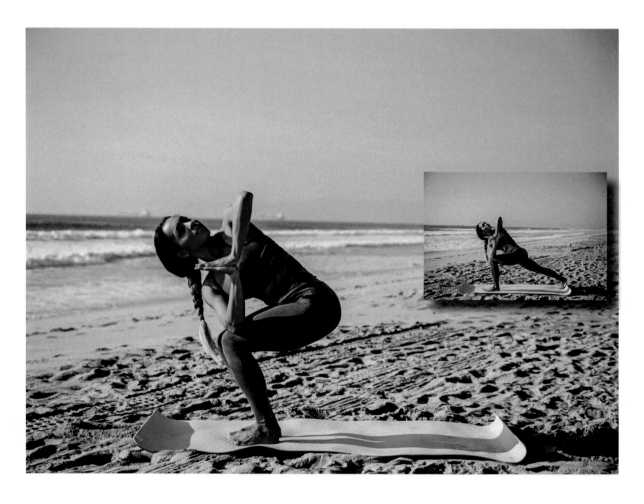

20. High Lunge

From revolved side angle in prayer pose, slowly lift your chest and arms up by using your abs. Arms go straight up to the sky, then tilt your pelvis forward, keeping the legs in a high lunge position. Keep chest open and breathe. Feel the weight equally distributed between both legs. Hold.

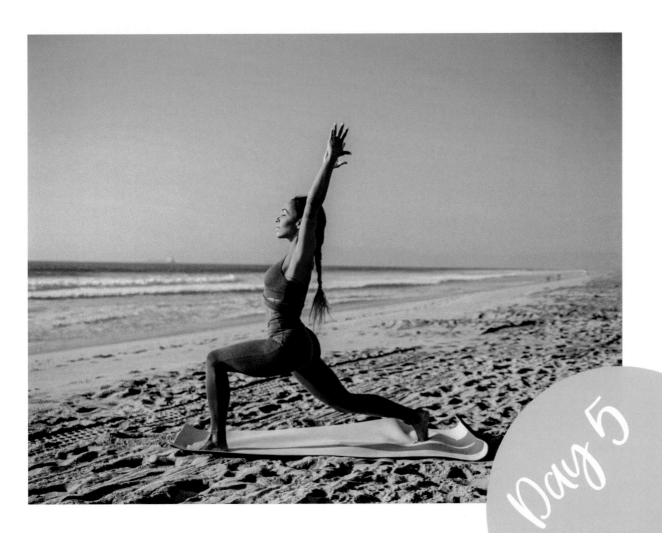

Day 5

21. Warrior 3

From high lunge, push off and fly! Lift up your back foot and keep both hips facing forward. Extend your arms and chest forward until they're parallel to the floor. Your back leg should also be parallel to the floor while you are in a straight line from back leg to the top of your head. Make sure your hips are leveled and not stacked. Feel all your muscles contract . . . and breathe!

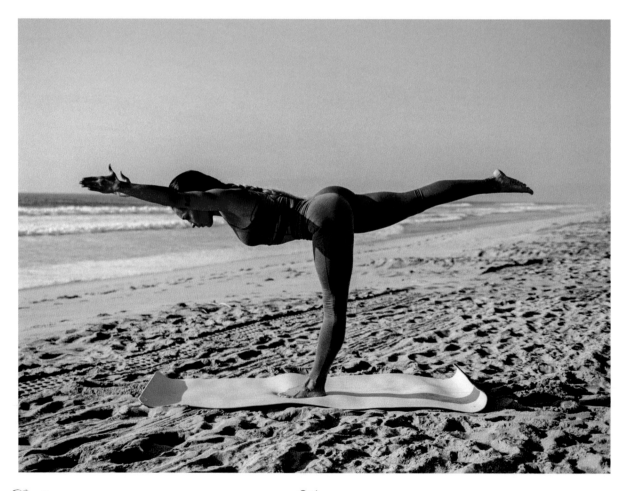

22. Standing Split

from Warrior 3, bring your arms down to the, floor framing the foot, and bend your whole upper body down so that your chest comes close to your thigh. Simultaneously lift the back leg as high as you can (it's ok to open the hips a bit here). Try to bring your forehead to your chin. Once you feel stable, grab your ankle with one hand, then both hands, instead of resting them on the ground. Breathe in and out of your nose and hold it as long as you can.

Switch sides

From standing split, lower the lifted leg down and have your feet meet each other on the mat, side-by-side. Relax into forward fold then bend your knees and lift up into chair pose (18). Repeat steps 19 - 22 on the left side. End in forward fold.

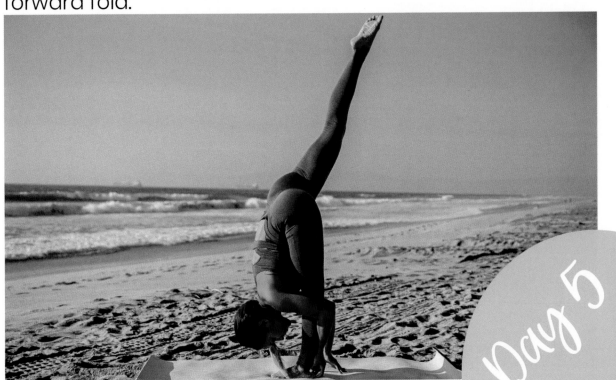

Day 5

82

23. Wrist Stretch

From forward fold, place your hands on the ground. Bend your knees and kneel to the on your mat. Sit up straight (no rounding your back) and keep your shoulders back and down (slightly retracted). Lift your arms forward and parallel to the ground. Move ONLY your hands in all directions while breathing . . . up, down, make a fist, open out to the sides, flip the palms inward, and so on. Continue motions while breathing for about a minute. You can sit cross-legged if the kneeling hurts your knees.

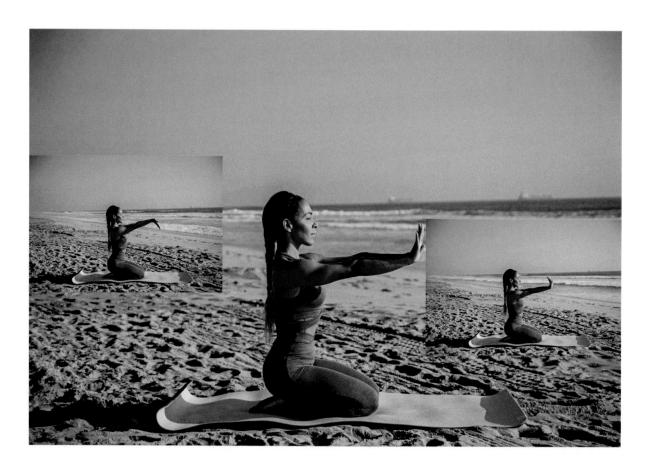

24. Cactus To Protraction

While still kneeling (or cross legged), open up both of your arms out to the side and as far back as possible. Open the chest and inhale while looking up to the sky (shoulder blades together). Next, go into opposition by bringing your chin to your chest, clasping your hands in front of you and outward (separating your shoulder blades). Your back is rounded here. Hallow out the belly and exhale! Go back and forth between the two about 10 times/10 breaths.

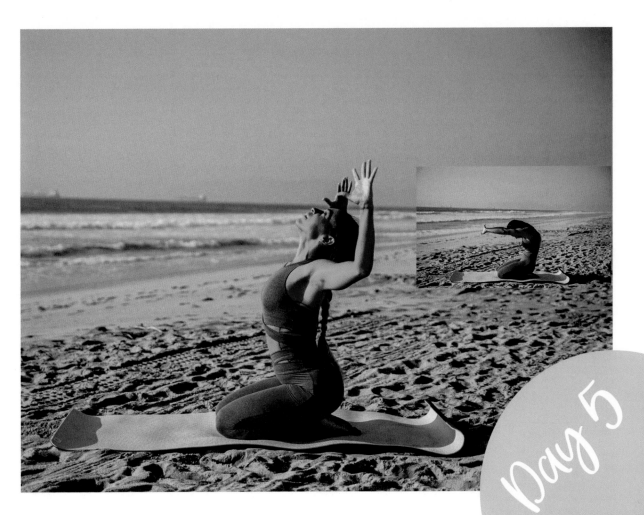

Day 5

25. Camel

Finally, lift your butt off your heels until your thighs and body are vertical. Go to your knees and place your hands behind you on your hips (as if you're putting them into back pockets). Look up and back as far as you can while keeping your hips forward and the length in your spine. Try not to collapse into it, but rather, lengthen up and back. Keeping the hips forward is key here. Squeeze your shoulder blades together. If you can see what's behind you, go ahead and touch your heels with the palms of your hands. Otherwise, stay where you are and breathe (5 breaths).

Come out slowly the same way you entered into the pose by putting your hands on the lower back and slowly pushing up.

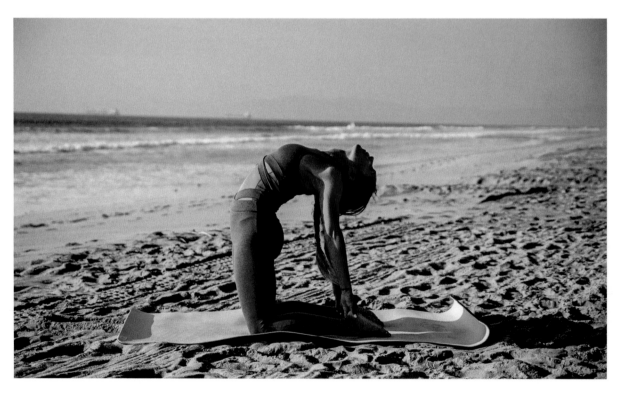

lay down on your mat and relax. YOU DID IT!

Day 5

Cucumber Salad
With Lemon Dressing

Awesome side dish to any meal! I also love having it in the middle of the day as a snack. Cucumber salads, most of the time, are preserved, unless you're in a restaurant that prepares it fresh. The added sweet corn gives it a great contrast to the sour dressing, which is something I just tried out one day and stuck with it because it was so yummy. The fact that cucumbers also contain fiber and are rich in water (and both of those assets promote digestion). makes it even more of a plus to have this along with your lunch or dinner. Or, by itself at any given time of the day... Little ingredients, lots of flavor. Little calories, lots of satisfaction.

Prep: 10min, Cook: 0min, Total Time: 10min

What You Need
(for 2 servings):

1 cucumber
½ small onion
½ a cup of sweet corn
salt
fresh ground pepper
fresh chopped Parsley

Optional Add ons: Another yummy add on would be a red, orange or yellow pepper!

Prepare:

1. Peel and chop up the cucumber in half, then small pieces of halfs.
2. place it into bowl and add Corn and chopped onion.
3. Add seasoning, (except parsley).
4. Straight into the bowl, add the dressing ingredients and mix well
5. Sprinkle the parsley on top.

Yummmmm!

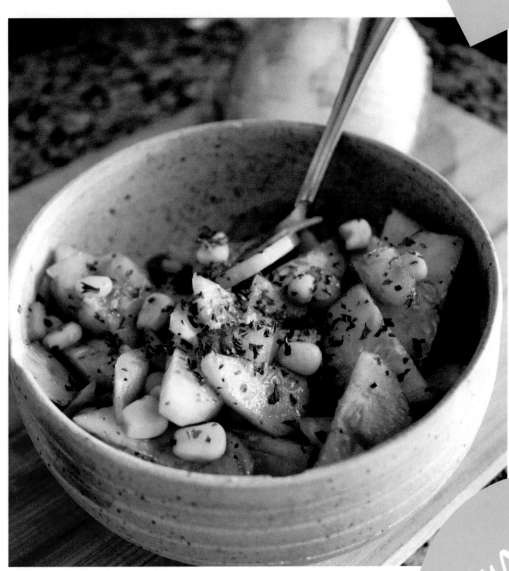

Day 5

Day 6

Run!

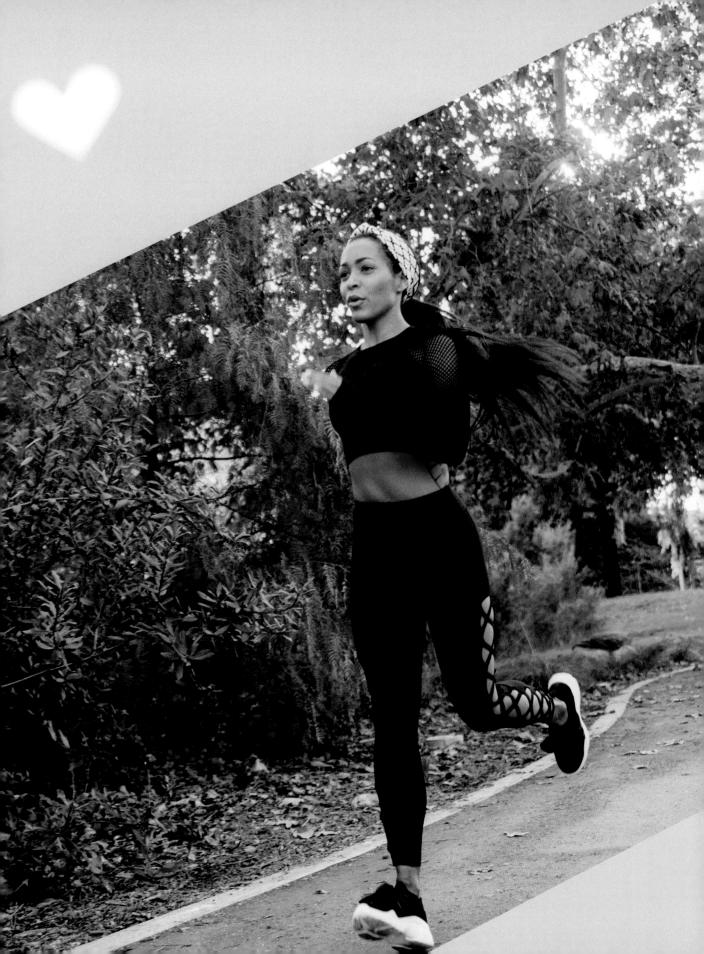

There are two types of people in this world: The Runners and the Non-Runners. Or it could be that you're a Runner who just doesn't run much because the thought of it is exhausting, but whenever you do get into that sprint, you feel amazing and powerful! I am that type. You may be the type to just absolutely dread it all together. Whichever type you are, be ready, because today we will RUN.

Since some of us are more advanced, while others are just getting back into working out, and some may just not ever run at all (unless there's an emergency), I have created three levels. All three levels require you to have about 45 minutes to yourself (no kids). If you're a full-time mommy, and if necessary, you can swap out this day with a different one in this guide and do this challenge when you can manage to get some help with the babies!!

TOTAL running time is only 25 minutes. Easy!

The motto today is (just like each time we jump into physical challenge), Don't Think About It: Just Do It! Remember that! The more you think about it, the harder it gets! This is a fact!!

Outdoors:

Treadmill

Level 1 Goal: 2miles
-Be sure to sprint at least 3 times
-Be sure your walking breaks don't exceed 2min

Level 2 Goal: 3miles
-Be sure to switch up the tempo as much as possible.
-Be sure your walking breaks don't exceed 2min

Level 3 Goal: 4miles
-Be sure to switch up the tempo as much as possible.
-Be sure your walking breaks don't exceed 1 min

Pace	Time	Speed lvl 1	Speed lvl 2	Speed lvl 3
Walk	4 min	3.5 mph	3.7 mph	4 mph
Jog	2 min	5.5 mph	6 mph	7 mph
Walk	1 min	3.5 mph	3.7 mph	4 mph
Run	2 min	7 mph	7.5 mph	8 mph
Walk	2 min	3.5 mph	3.7 mph	4 mph
Jog	2 min	5.5 mph	6 mph	7 mph
Sprint	30 sec	8 mph	9.5 mph	11 mph
Walk	2 min	3.5 mph	3.7 mph	4 mph
Jog	1 min	5.5 mph	6 mph	7 mph
Run	2 min	7 mph	3.7 mph	8 mph
Walk	3 min	3.5 mph	3.7 mph	4 mph
Sprint	30 sec	8 mph	9.5 mph	11 mph
Walk	2 min	3.5 mph	3.7 mph	4 mph
Cooldown	1 min	2.2 mph	2.8 mph	3 mph

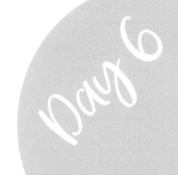

Day 6

Brown Rice Spaghetti
With Tomato & Pesto

Prep:5min, Cook:10min, Total Time:15min

What You Need (for 2 servings)
2 tablespoons of green pesto
olive oil
2 garlic cloves
brown rice spaghetti
1. Can of diced tomatoes

green basil pesto
salt & pepper
paprika powder
soy sauce
2 tablespoons of shredded
parmesan cheese
(chili powder if you
like it spicey)

Prepare:
1. Boil the pasta for 8-10min.
2. While pasta is boiling, in a pan heat up 2 tablespoons of olive oil.
3. Peel and slice up garlic cloves, then saute them in medium heat for about 3min.
4. Add the whole can of diced tomatoes.
2. Season generously with salt, pepper, paprika and soy sauce (and chili).
4. Drain the pasta and place it into the pan with the tomato mix.
5. Add pesto and cheese, then stir everything.
6. Serve Hot.

FOOD OF THE DAY

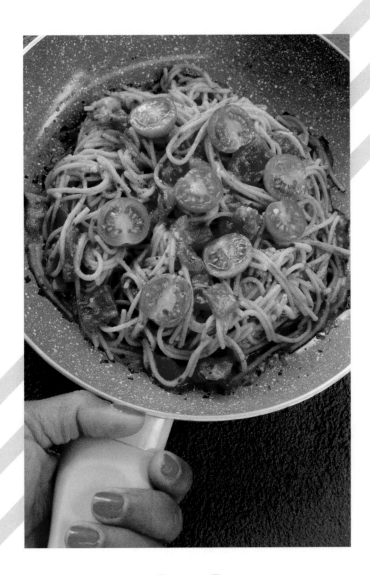

Day 6

Day 7

Clean House

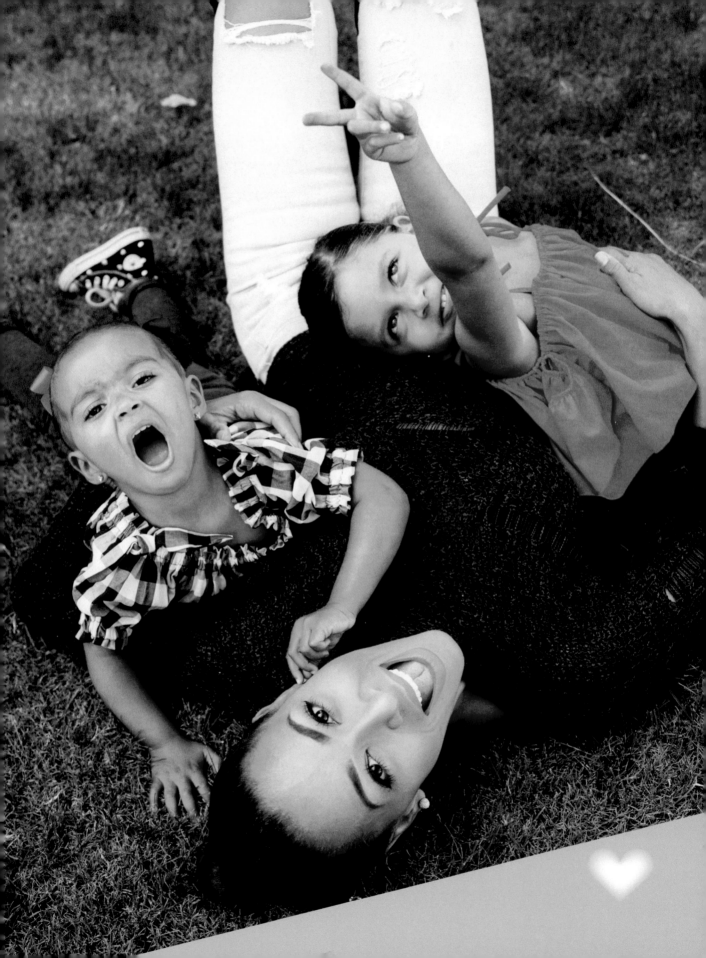

Hello, Gorgeous! I grant you a break from working out today, unless you're a warrior and want to break into a sweat (you can ALWAYS add on to this guide with whatever you feel does your body good). I personally take some days off during the week just because I have enough things to do!! Also, because it does the body good to recover every few days — especially after that RUN we had yesterday! So, let's focus on something else that is going to have a major effect on our mood and well-being!

It's Cleaning time! And, yes, it can be a workout to clean, if you don't have a housekeeper!! Even doing the laundry, especially if you have kids, can be a LOT! Like my song "Love my Life" says: "The laundry's piling up the ceiling." I wasn't lying! LOL

First things first: MAKE YOUR BED! I make mine every single day, and you may too, but if you don't, let this be the first thing you do after getting out that bed! It always sets the mood for me, even if the rest of the house is a mess. It does something and sends me off into the day with good vibes.

Whenever you take your time for this challenge today, start with the little things and work your way towards the major "messes" in the house In my case it's always my closet (shrugs). I just can't keep my closet nice and neat … Ever! I also own way too many things I don't need, so getting rid of clothes and toys, like once every other month, is something I had to make a habit of doing! Some of us may be very organized, neat freaks, but chances are, if you're a mom without a housekeeper, your house is always in need of straightening up! ALWAYS. The minute you finish the dishes, there is a mess in the kids room, the second you vacuum, there is clean laundry that needs to be folded and the trash that needs to be taken out. After that, it's time to eat again and, boom, another mess has suddenly occurred, especially after cooking (see Food of the Day). 😉 With kids running around, my entire living room area has turned into a playroom and the amount of toys (and even food leftovers) I find under my couch sometimes is insane! I get irritated sometimes when people ask me what I've been doing all day, because . . . DUH! I've been doing "Mom Life" stuff, like taking care of the household!! IT JUST NEVER ENDS!

So, let's get to it! And also remember, when you're at it, ALLOW YOUR KIDS TO TAKE PART. My babies love when I do something they can help with. Turn the TV off for a while and play some music. Open all your blinds and let the daylight in! Once you've taken care of the basics, like dishes and laundry, find some time to organize an area in your space. It may be your closet (like in my case) or your kids closet, or a desk, or your kitchen table. Unfortunately, my kitchen table is like a drop-off station for all unnecessary items and unopened mail. Shaking My Head (SMH).

Day 7

It takes time to get organized, so take the time! Even if you don't get everything done, just like with all your other goals in life, take it step by step! A little progress counts! And I had to learn that. I used to think, "Oh, I don't have enough time now to do all that. I gotta be somewhere in 2 hours." I wouldn't touch anything and I'd put it off until "the next time." The key is to just start though! You can do a lot in one hour if you don't let distractions get in your way.

The goal for today is to have at least one bag of things/toys/clothes that's a giveaway bag! Nothing but positive comes from letting go of clutter. Just like a bad relationship, let go and make room for new and better things in your world.

Homemade Tuna Salad

FOOD OF THE DAY

Funny story: I used to order tuna salad sandwiches at the deli in New York and always wondered how they were made. I followed my taste buds, and one day I started making tuna salad at home just mixing the different ingredients I could taste (without checking online for a recipe)! Afterwards, I researched and found that most tuna salads contained exactly what I had guessed, except the mustard I used (which gives it the spice I love). Also, most other recipes I found had celery instead of onions, but try it my way and see if you like it! I think it's the BOMB!

Prep:8 min Cook:0 min Total Time:8 min

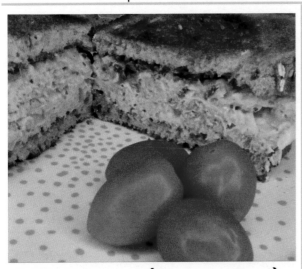

What you Need (For 2 portions):
2 cans of tuna in water
1 dill pickle
½ small onion
2 tbsp of mayonnaise
1 tbsp of mustard (any kind you like)
garlic powder
salt & pepper

Prepare:
Place all the tuna into a bowl
Chop up the onion and the pickle in tiny pieces (as small as possible!)
Add Mayo and mustard sprinkle with Garlic powder, Salt and Pepper
stir well (with a fork)
Enjoy on Whole wheat Toast or with your choice of crackers

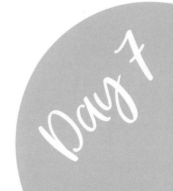

Day 7

Day 8

Clear Your Mind

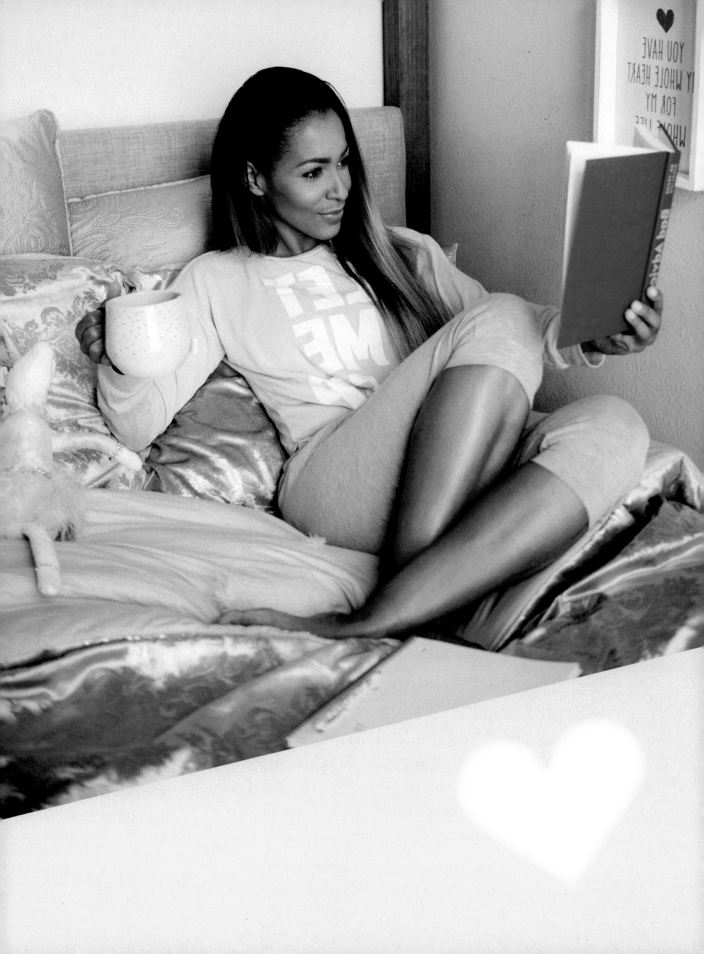

Happy Day 8! One week has gone by and you did it! If you've been dedicated and open to these new and different approaches to your days, you rock, and now it's going to be a piece of cake to continue, even though we're not even halfway there. It may be an even better experience if you have adjusted the rest of your days around this Day 8 challenge. What this means is that you've gone past the two hours that these activities/workouts and recipes require.

Maybe you've applied some elements of certain days in this book into your everyday life. Perhaps you've done the yoga flow I included into this challenge every day since Yoga Day. Or maybe you've just done exactly what was listed for each day as of now. Whatever it is, you are on your way to becoming a better and more at-ease you — someone who can enjoy each day of your life, no matter your circumstances.

After cleaning house yesterday, we are focusing on our **mind** today. Going for a power walk (even if you're pushing a stroller) should be a definite activity today. Make that your number one activity today! It can be so rejuvenating. I always choose to walk somewhere instead of driving if it's within a one mile radius. Yes, I live in California and weather plays a big part, but unless it's pouring outside, there are no excuses. Get cozy in warm clothes if it's cold where you are. Getting fresh air is a must!! Having two babies, I often grab one and put her on my back (carrier), and push the other one in the stroller. It's amazing how many people stop and give me props, firing me up, when they see me! Those times will soon be over, as my girls are growing up way too fast. 😌 Having a clear mind is equally as important as eating right or working out. If your mind is cluttered with things because you have a lot to do and you are overwhelmed by all of it, you get stressed out — and so do I. But there are things you can do to reduce the stress. We are doing one of the stress reducers today. And that is, **Writing down a To-Do checklist**. Make this your second task! I used to always just keep my list in my head, but that caused my mind to get so swamped that it had a huge effect on my moods. And I am still struggling to keep a calendar. Yeah, like I said, I ain't perfect. I still work on taking my own advice a lot, so we are all in this together. But as I'm learning and sharing, I just feel it all coming together more and more and the positivity is overflowing — at least in my house! WE GOT THIS.Now, back to the **mind**.

Day 8

If it is cluttered with unimportant, insignificant things like opinions of others or what this or that person had to say about you or even straight gossip, there is another list I'm going to have you start writing today while we're at it, and that is your list of **GOALS**. And it may only be one, or it may be two or five. But if you have a hard time trying to find a goal, we have somewhat of a problem.

If your goal is to be "happy," I encourage you to start thinking about the things that make you happy. Getting closer to those things would be your goals. And if you just don't know what would make you happy, think of the time in your life you were the happiest. What was it about during that time that made you happy? Is it being a child again and not having the worries of an adult — like bills? Well, there is no way to go back to that or change the fact that you are an adult and you have bills to pay and other things to take care of. How about working towards finding ways to not have to   worry about your bills? I know, it's something we all want, and easier said than done. But you just have to understand that something like "Getting Money" is not going to come overnight. However, it will never come if you don't start making moves. I'm preaching common knowledge here, I know, but I have come to the realization that complaining is not going to change anything. The only thing that can change things in your life are your actions, and you taking initiative and control over your life. Now, If it is a person you think of when you think of your happiest times, figure out why they made you happy.

A little story: This hits home for me, because I recall talking to my therapist when I was going through my last breakup about nothing else being able to make me feel the way that person made me feel. My therapist then challenged me to find other things that made me feel those happy feelings. There was nothing. At least that is what I thought. However, I tried really hard to take that challenge seriously. I sat down and started thinking about what it really was that made me so happy with that person. In the end I figured out that there was only one other thing in life that had ever given me that feeling, that rush of happiness, that feeling of just really LIVING, and it was being creative. It was getting lost in my art (my music) by bringing something alive that will exist forever, even if only my ears heard it now.

Besides that, I realized that the person had made me enjoy the "regular" things in life. And yes, I enjoyed them when I was with him, but I realized the things we used to do together I was definitely able to do alone or with someone else, except I had never enjoyed those things as much alone or with anyone else. But why wasn't this possible? It turns out it IS possible. I had to learn how to

BE in the moment — realizing that all we have is now. A beautiful beach is still beautiful when you're alone. My problem was I never put my focus on the beach, but on that person, and it was almost like I wanted him to enjoy it more than me. Seeing him enjoy it made me happy. Trying to enjoy a place or an activity or a song (or whatever it may have been) wasn't something I was sure I knew how to do, but I worked hard on putting my focus on the things we used to do and love, and off of him. I started making myself aware of my surroundings and the things I do every day. Awareness had really become a major key in my life whether it's body awareness or the awareness of self and what was around me.

And this is exactly what I have taken from that relationship; the ability to enjoy things that are happening now, "regular" things. It almost feels like it was a lesson to help me enjoy life, even when things are hard and when nothing is going right. You still have to make sure that you make everyday count.

Being surrounded by

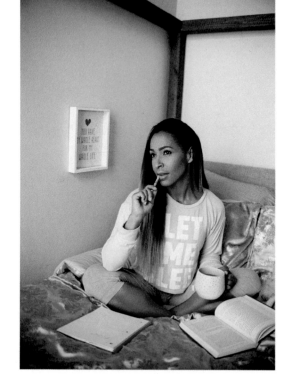

great people is always a good thing. Feeling loved and uplifted is reviving in many ways, but being alone and feeling FULL is the most amazing place to be. And I'm speaking from experience. It feels like nothing can break you. As a matter of fact, CAN'T NOTHING BREAK YOU. It is so important to me to spend time with myself these days, and myself a lot of times is me and my girls (and they are pretty much me). LOL

So we've got our lists, and we've got the power walk. Now let's eat!

Day 8

Apfel Muesli
(Apples and Oats)

When you wake up in the morning, the first foods you should want to put into your system are fresh foods. And by fresh I mean uncooked! From my childhood I remember loving this dish, which I got from my mother, who would make it for me and my sisters in less than 10 minutes. It's easy, simple, healthy, and most importantly, yummy! Nowadays, my kids and I love having this for breakfast, which is not necessarily only a breakfast meal. But I guess the oatmeal and the orange juice puts it into the breakfast category, as well as the fact that it is delicious with a cup of coffee or tea! This is one of those dishes that you cannot stop eating after you take the first bite.

Prep: 8 min Cook: 0 min Total time: 8 min

Prepare:
1. Peel the apple entirely
2. Shred it into bowl, down to the core
3. Add oatmeal (not cooked) and raisins
4. Chop up the almonds and add those
5. Add orange juice and stir
6. Top with cinnamon to your liking

What You Need (for 2 servings):
1 Large Apple
1 ½ cup of old fashioned oatmeal
⅓ cup of almonds
⅓ cup full of raisins
cinamon
cup of orange juice (not from concentrate)

Add ons:
My mother used to always put coconut flakes on it, which gave it an amazing twist. You can also mix in any kind of dried or fresh fruit, like banana or berries, to add more flavor I love a spritz of lemon juice (but I'm sure most kids like it rather sweet), so I keep that for myself! 😉

FOOD OF THE DAY

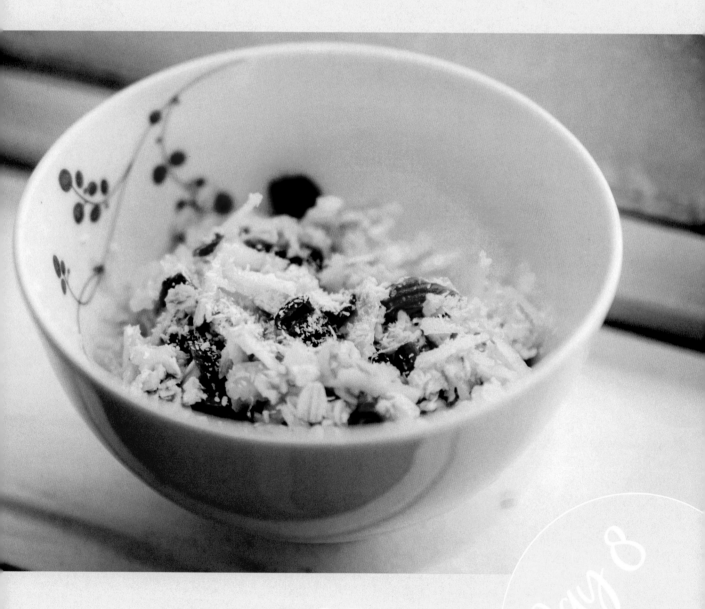

Day 8

♥

Day 9

The Good Medium

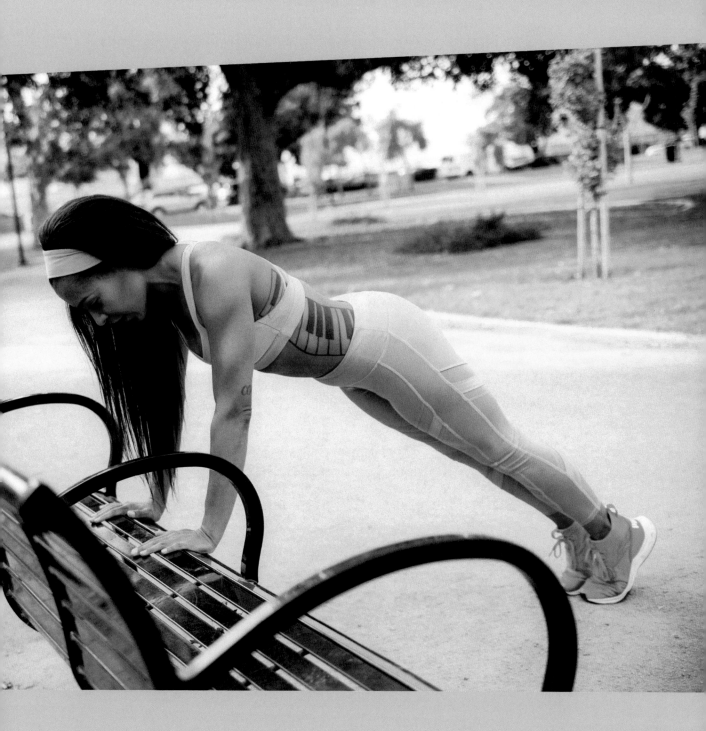

"Go Hard or Go Home" is something I definitely do *not* live by. I totally believe, "A little goes a long way." By now you've gotten a pretty decent preview of how I like to approach my workout regimen. In my life, when it comes to regularity vs. diversity, diversity definitely wins. And it wasn't always like that. I touched on this in one of the previous chapters, but I used to ALWAYS do the same workout. I did the same kind of high intensity cardio, which produced the same kind of sweat and the same kind of exhaustion in the end. Yes, I was in okay shape, but was I feeling my best? No! I've never felt as good as I do now that I don't put that pressure on myself that I have to have a certain amount of calories burned every time I workout! I honestly don't even weigh myself much. Every now and then I step on the scale just out of curiosity, but whatever the numbers say, I couldn't care less. I used to be scared of what I might possibly see. All I always wanted, becoming an adult, was to weigh under 60 kg (132lbs, in Germany we go by kilo). But I've come to realize that 132lbs is just an unrealistic weight for my height (5'6) and muscular body type. Nowadays I'm around 140lbs and I don't even know what exactly that is in kilo, nor do I care. It's all about how I feel! And I feel

GOOD. 😊

I want you to achieve this satisfaction as well, and while my book isn't so much about losing weight, but more about feeling good in your skin and your everyday life, we all know when you look better, you feel better.

Sooo! Today we are back at it with the physical work. But it will be fairly easy. We are not going crazy with it but lets get a good 30 minutes in! Again, if you do have a gym available and are "kids free," HIT IT! But you can also do this at home with the babies in the background, as I do a lot of the times! It's a great day for some abs and arm exercises!

What you need:
2 Light Dumbbells
(5-8 lbs)

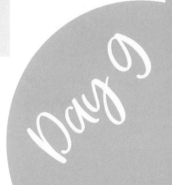
Day 9

1.Plank.

Start in a Plank position and hold for 1 min. Then start tapping your shoulders --still in plank (right hand left shoulder, left hand right shoulder.. And so on) Tap your shoulders at least 30 times.

2.V-Sit Shoulder press.

Sit on floor with your knees bent, hold a dumbbell in each hand by hips. Lean back 45 degrees and lift your feet (shins parallel to floor). Keep your posture and start extending your arms up above head 20 times

3.Jackknive Crunches

Lay flat on your back holding dumbbells in hands (no dumbbells for beginners). Lift and lower legs straight while lifting and lowering arms straight (above head). Do it 10-15 times. Important: Keep your lower back flat on the floor at all times.

4.Russian Twist.

Sit on the floor with your knees bent. Lean back (45 degree angle) and lift your feet (shins should be parallel to the floor). Beginners can do this one without dumbbells and let your feet touch the ground. Otherwise, hold the dumbbells and twist left and right 10-15 times each.

5.Push-Ups:

Start in plank position, Hands underneath your shoulders, Lower your body down, but Don't touch the floor, keep your ellbows in and close to the body, do not round your back and keep your hips low and in a straight line with the rest of your body, push up and repeat 10-15 times
(if you're a beginner, do the same move on your knees)

6.Tricep Dips

Sit on the floor with knees bent and with feet touching the floor. Place your hands next to your hips on the floor and lift up your butt. Bendi your elbows (minimal bend) and then straighten. Repeat 10-15 times. If you are more advanced, find a higher surface, such as a chair, bench or table and GO FOR IT! Make sure your hips stay close to the chair, bench or table.

Go back to the beginning and repeat exercises 1-6. Three rounds total.
Note: All of these can be done without dumbbells for an easier option.

Day 9

MI Healthy Peaches & Cream SHAKE
(blender required)

I just recently started making shakes at home after i finally purchased a blender, For years i would just always go get a jamba juice or something of that sort, but it is so easy and cheaper AND more exciting when you can create your own! Like with my salads i like to experiment with different fruit and juices . Here is one of my favorite shakes to make at home. My favorite time to have it is after a workout!!

What you need (for one shake):

½ cup of cashews
½ cup of Low-fat Greek yogurt
1 tablespoon Chia seeds
1 cup of frozen peaches
1 cup of water
½ teaspoon of cinnamon
1 tablespoon honey or agave syrup
2 tablespoons of vanilla protein powder (optional)

Prepare:

Put everything into the blender and blend thoroughly!

DONE!

FOOD OF THE DAY

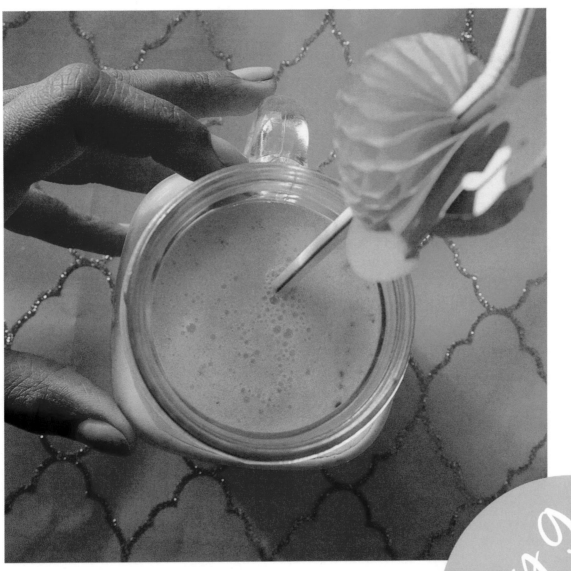

Day 9

Day 10

GO IN

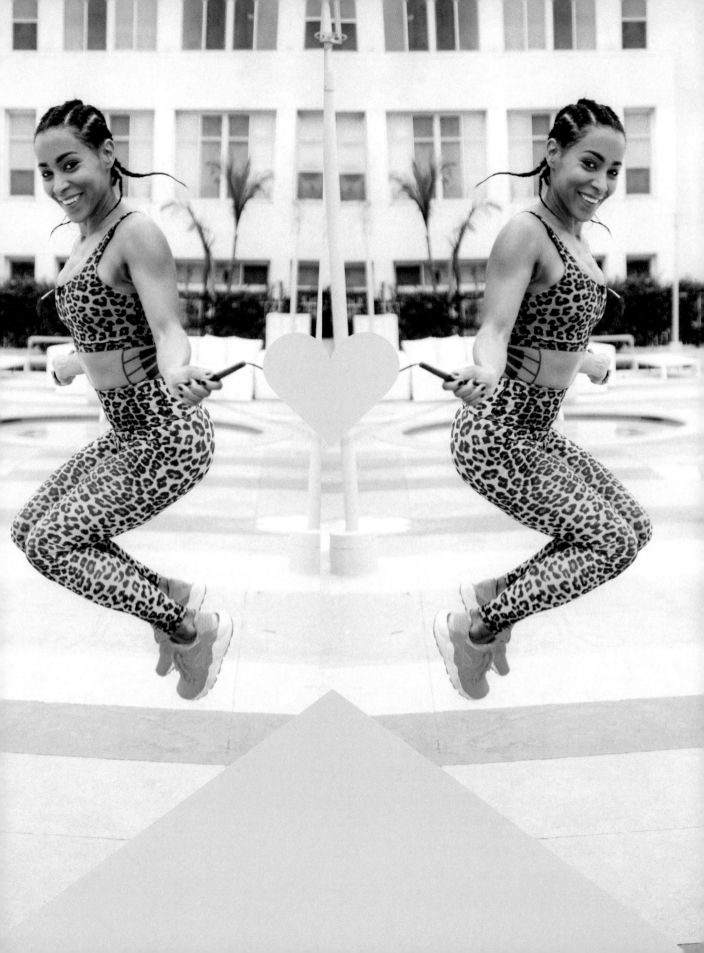

Hello, Queen! If it's morning, **Think Positive** vibes only! If it's the afternoon, **Think Positive** vibes only! If it's evening, **Think Positive** vibes only! I know, I know: Things happen around us all the time that make us feel unrelaxed or irritated, but you are you, and those things won't change a thing about that! Do me a favor and don't compare yourself to others today – OR ANY DAY – never, ever again! Whatever may be bothering you — whether it's a fight you had with a friend or with your significant other (or maybe you're feeling stressed with work), push that to the side for a little while. I am telling you, if you force yourself to step away from something for a while then come back to it, chances are your feelings will change — especially if you get a workout in!

Much like on our Day 2, we are going to really get it in today! So if you can, get it out of the way in the morning! I am way more motivated to work out in the morning than I am in the evening. It may be different for you, but when I finish my workout early, I'm always in a way better mood and I don't have to think about it for the rest of the day. All I do is FEEL GOOD!

I mean, come on. What is an hour out of your day? You must fall in love with taking care of yourself — your Body. Mind and Spirit. Yeah, I've read that somewhere, but it is so true. The only way things will change for the better is if you to learn how to enjoy the process and the progress.

The FULL Body routine from Day 2 is a great exercise to repeat today! Don't forget to also do your

30 minutes of cardio! You can get on the Treadmill (from day 6), or if you have kids and no gym, jump rope (from Day 3)! Make it work, and remember to *really* push yourself on our Pink days! We don't do a lot of these days, so we have to make sure to go ALL Out! You can even extend the workout if you have it in you! Today, you need to feel complete exhaustion!

MOMMY TIP

If you have an infant, you have plenty of time (during his/her nap) to get into a quick sweat! And yes, young moms, scheduling your workouts within your child's nap is key and soooo totally possible — even if they may nap for only 20 minutes sometimes. You can do something in 20! Choose to move your body before you do anything else. You will be glad afterwards!

Day 10

Bread And Things

In Germany, where i was born, people eat a lot of bread, and yes all we hear all the time is how bad bread is for you, but truth is, if you choose the right kind of bread, it is actually not so bad for you! Choose a bread high in Fiber and do not eat White bread! At least not a lot. Ill have it sometimes when im at a barbecue and eat a hot dog bun or at the cheesecake factory when the bread comes out and i'm starving, but try to always go for the dark!! And when you buy bread for the house look at the ingredients! A lot of time the bread looks dark but actually isn't! Here in America it has been a struggle finding those breads i grew up eating. Fresh Whole grain loafs? Most people don't even buy bread at bakeries, but in the supermarket where all they have is packaged fake whole wheat breads. Anyway, where I'm from we don't have the term "Dinner", instead its called: "Abend Brot" = "Evening Bread" would be the exact translation. The reason behind it is that many people simply eat bread with yummy things on it. Toppings. One can get very creative here! And don't be afraid to try something new. I chose to always have something fresh on my bread! Try it!

Prep: 5min, Cook: 0min, Total Time: 5min

What you need:
4 Slices of Whole grain bread (best to buy it fresh from a bakery)

½ avocado

3 grape tomatoes

Hummus (any kind you like)

1/4th of a Cucumber/ or 1 Persian Cucumber

Peanut butter Raw (just peanuts)

½ Banana

Nutella/ or a different kind of Hazelnut spread

3 strawberries

Prepare:
1. Place all 4 pieces of bread onto a big plate or cutting board.
2. Get creative! Spread the base (avocado, hummus, PB, nutella) onto each piece of bread in the amount you like.
3. cut up the toppings (Tomatoes, cucumber, banana, strawberries)
4. arrange on each assignd bread.
5. sprinkle salt and pepper onto the cucumber and tomatoes

FOOD OF THE DAY

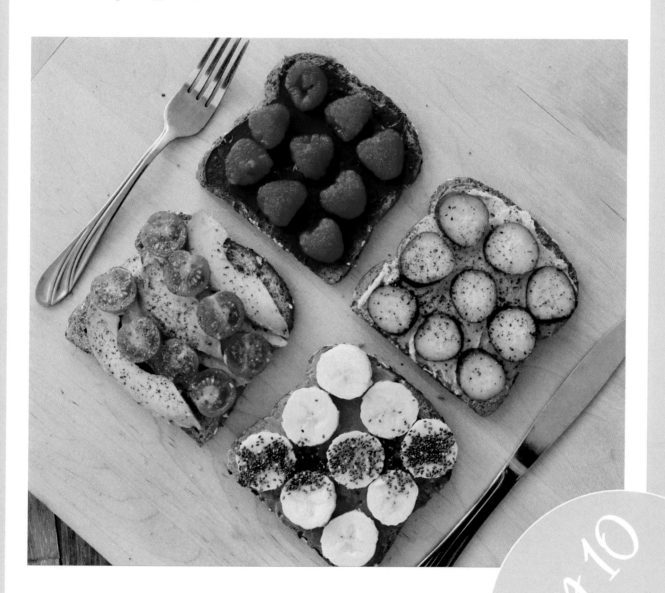

Day 10

Day 11

It's a Feast!

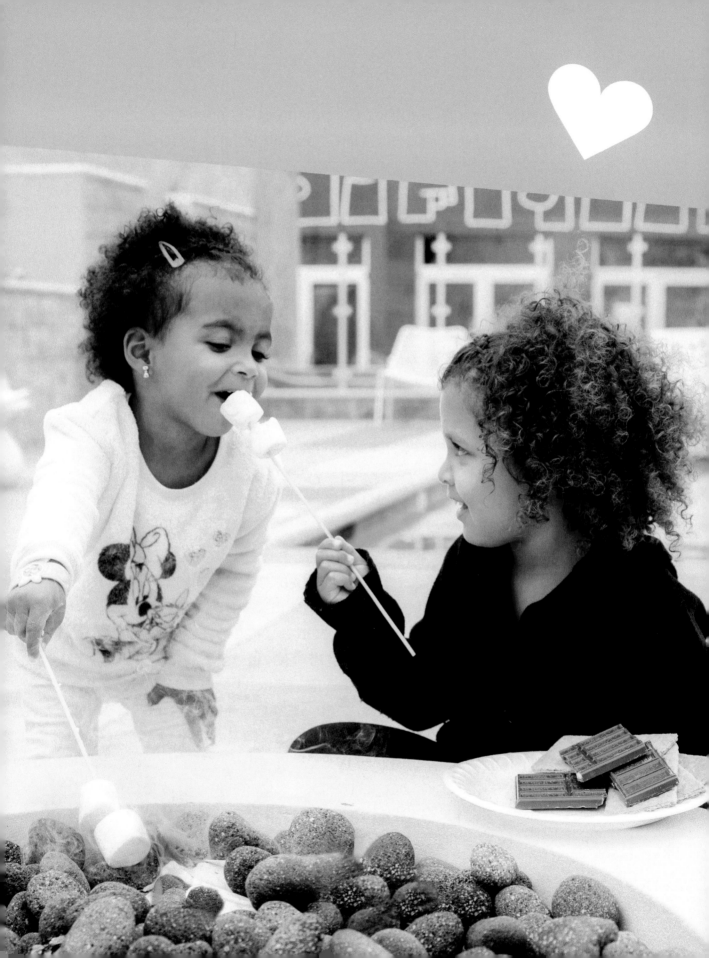

Guess what? I almost wanted to call this "Cheat Day," but I'm NOT. You want to know why? Because in my world there are no cheat days, simply because I never restrict myself from anything, so it's never "cheating" when I eat something high in calories or fat, or even processed (although most processed foods really are just bad for you). The main thing you should be trying to accomplish is *not wanting them all the time*. I have definitely gotten to that point, which feels great, because when you follow a certain life-style you crave different kinds of foods! Yes, you may say I grew up in Germany - eating differently, which is true, but what's the matter with being open to trying new things? What I know is that it becomes easier to eat healthy (mostly), when you change not only the food intake, but all of the other things I talk about in this book, especially your mind!

With this guide I have not given you a diet plan or anything to stick to or cut out completely, on purpose. As a matter of fact, people have this misconception (especially on my food page on Instagram @mi_dishes) that I ONLY eat "health foods," which is not the case and even in this guide I have some indulging, yummy recipes that are higher in calories or fat. But it is what I need to have every now and again to feel happy. It is also why some of my workout days (PINK days) are meant to be taken seriously. I take them very serious and so should you. If you want to indulge every now and then, like me, you must work hard! It's about BALANCE! Restrictions in my diet used to be my killer! If you just can't have something, you want it even more — so have less of it instead.

Again, I never feel like I'm on a diet, and you shouldn't either. Yes, some days we say "No" to things, but it's because we really don't want them. And yes, I'm speaking for us now. You are pretty much becoming family through this process. 😉😊 I mean, I see my daughters eat pizza, and sure, most of the time I'm tempted to get me a slice (and sometimes I do), but most times I will just have a couple of bites from their slice because even though I could totally eat my own slice, I don't want the feeling I get when I eat bad. It is not hard to say "No" to something you don't want. Your mouth and your mind may want it in that moment,

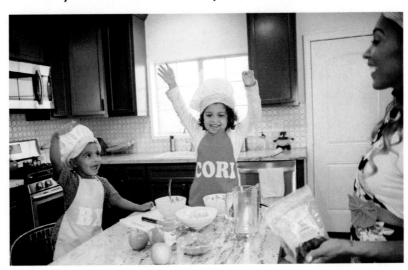

Day 11

but your body sure doesn't. It's as simple as that. Yes, we talked about being in the moment and enjoying what you love, but when it comes to your eating habits, let's also keep the moments in mind that are to come after you finish your fried foods. If you love your body, you simply don't want to feed it BS all the time. If you are learning to love it by trying something different (like following this guide), YOU GO, GIRL!

And today, I have two recipes that I think will make your day perfect!

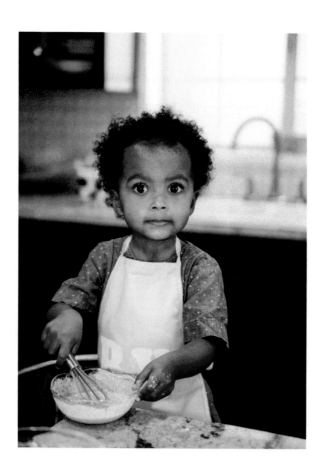

Healthy Snacks Suggestions

I always keep some of these in the house:

Baby Carrots

Persian cucumbers (cut up and sprinkle with salt)

Nuts

Blue corn tortilla chips and salsa

Dried fruits like cranberries/apricots

Fresh berries

Apples

Pretzels and Hummus

Low-fat plain Greek yogurt (Add honey)

BAMBA Peanut snack –from Trader Joes

Date and peanut bar–from Trader Joes

Animal crackers

Dark chocolate

Bananas

Baked Chips

Popcorn (skinny pop)

MOMMY TIP

If your kids are old enough, tell them the effect that eating too much junk and candy or chips can have on their stomach and their teeth. My kids are four and two (as I'm writing this book), which are good ages where they understand my reasoning. My daughter Cori LOVES sweets, especially chocolate, but she will take a few pieces and then pass it over to me because she knows if she eats the whole bar her tummy may start hurting! She knows from experience, and because mommy taught her! I have made things clear to my kids from the beginning, and they are learning about "good" and "bad" foods. It's amazing how my oldest will tell me she wants to have something healthy after finishing her ice cream. I feel like patting myself on the back whenever that happens!

Day 11

Pancakes.

When i first came to America i had to get used to 'fluffy' pancakes that soak up all the syrup and end up being a mess of sweet sludge. 'Pancake mix' was something i had never heard of. I only knew Pancakes from scratch, Pancakes the german way! It's almost like crepe' but better, in my opinion at least :-). And you have the option to use whole wheat or rye flour which makes it a higher fiber meal. Another super quick dish to make in the morning when your kids are impatient for their first bites of the day. Combine it with any fruit and it will not only taste amazing but also make a super pretty plate and you know how kids are when it comes to presentation.

FOOD OF THE DAY 1

Prepare:
1. Add flour into a bowl.
2. Whisk eggs and milk into it.
3. Add sugar.
4. Pour 1 cup of the mix into medium-heated vegetable oil pan.
5. Cook for 1-2 minutes on each side until slightly brown.
6. Serve on a plate and add more cinnamon and brown sugar to your liking.
7. Serve with apple sauce on the side or any fruit of your choice.

What You Need (4 servings):
2 eggs
3 cups of flour (whole wheat for a healthier choice)
3 tablespoons of brown sugar
2 cups of milk (any kind you like)
vegetable oil for the pan
applesauce for dipping
cinnamon sprinkle

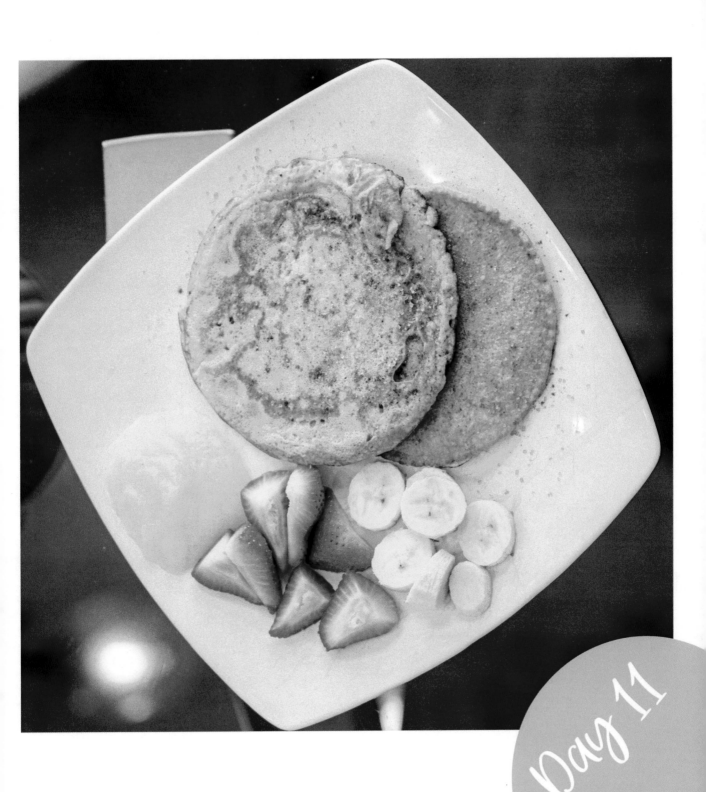

Day 11

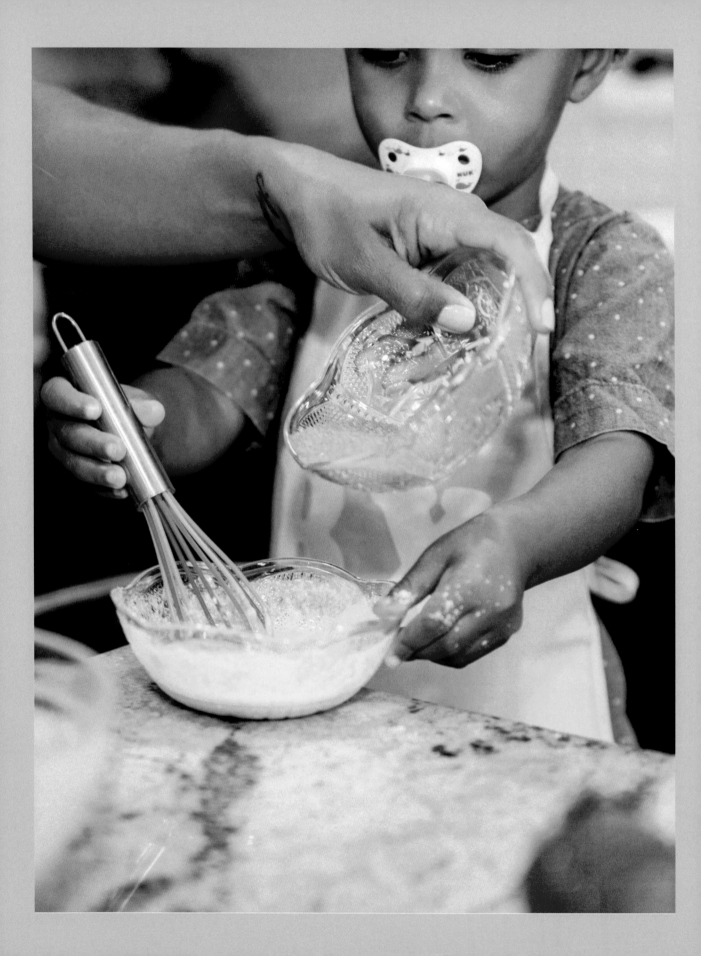

My day 11 does not include any working out — just because we need a break! And that is okay!

Get some snacks that you like. Try some snacks off my list on page 130 if you want to keep it on the healthy side, or I grant you permission to have your favorite junk food today. It's okay, as long as you don't have it again tomorrow!

And remember, you don't have to eat a lot today if you don't feel like you want it. You are also welcome to swap the day (for another day within the week) if today's choices don't suit you. What is important also is that if you do eat a lot today, don't have any negative thoughts afterwards. Don't regret it, and don't say, "I shouldn't have." Know that it's OKAY, because we don't have feast day everyday.

My suggestion for a yummy dinner may not be the healthiest, but I promise it's ahhhhmazing and you deserve it!

Turkey Chili

The "MI" stems from "MI_Dishes" which is my Insta food page. Originally the MI is taken from my first name "AMI," which is what my close family have called me all my life. Online, with the @ in front of it, it reads "@MI," which I thought was cool. This dish can be made spicy or mild. I love spicy foods and being that this is chili, you would probably assume it should be. But since I had my girls, I always have to cook mild and add the spice later on, which is completely doable! Kids love dipping bread into this yummy dish. I like to simply have a bit of sour cream and jalapeños on top.

Prepare:

1. In a large pot, heat up olive oil and sauté chopped onion and sliced garlic for 1-2 minutes on med-high heat.
2. Chop up the pepper and add into pot. Cook another 2 minutes.
3. Add ground turkey and cook while stirring for about 5-6 minutes.
4. Add salt& pepper
5. Add beans and a can of tomato sauce and diced tomato.
6. Add sugar, chili powder and soy sauce.
7. Cover with lid and cook on medium heat for about 15 minutes (stir occasionally). If it's too thick, add a bit of water.
8. Serve with a tablespoon of sour cream and shredded cheddar cheese and jalapeños if you like.
9. Add a ton of hot sauce of your choice (optional).

FOOD OF THE DAY 2

Prep: 5 min, Cook: 25 min, Total Time:30 min

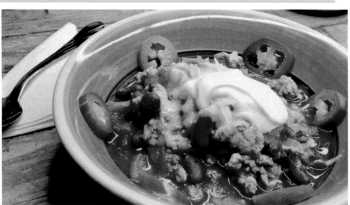

What you need (Serves about 6):

1 lb ground turkey
1 can of tomato sauce 15oz
1 can of diced tomato 15oz
1 can of dark red kidney beans 15oz
1 medium sized onion
2 sliced garlic cloves
1 red, yellow or orange pepper
1 tablespoon chili powder
1 tablespoon of brown sugar
2 tablespoon of soy sauce
1 tablespoon of salt
1 tablespoon of black pepper
3 tablespoons olive oil

For serving:
sour cream
shredded
cheese
jalapeños

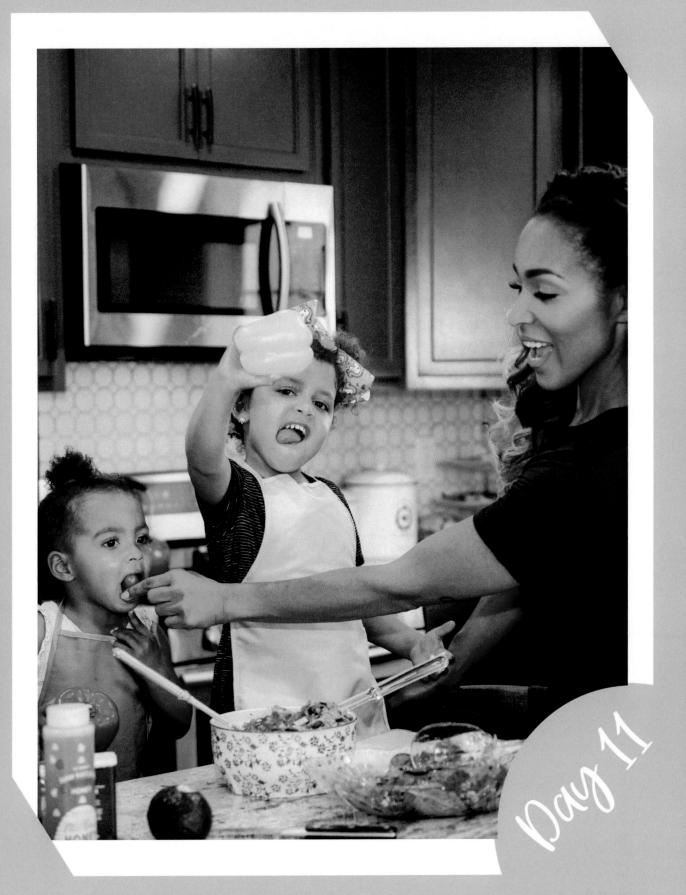

Day 12

Yogi Day

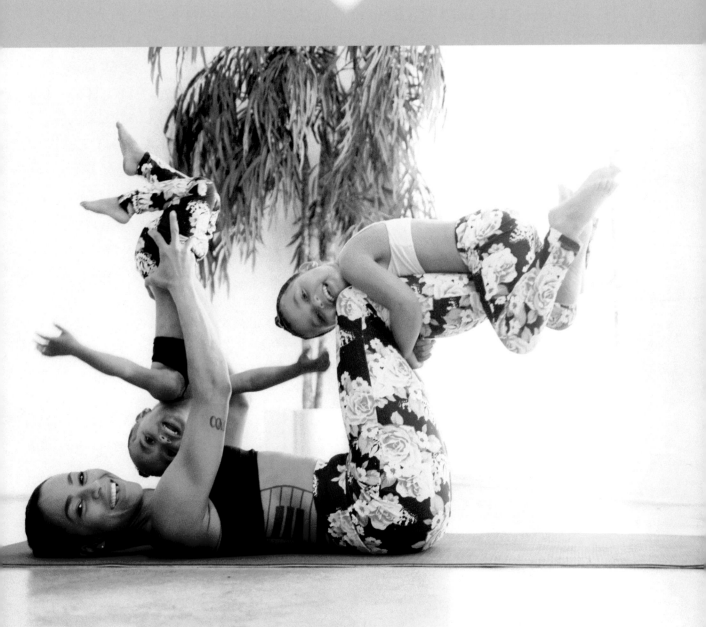

Rise and Shine! Even when the sun doesn't shine, YOU MUST! 😏 Remember that!

If you're not a morning person, you can still find a morning ritual that you really enjoy. For me it's getting my coffee, sitting by a window, and drinking it in silence (after I make breakfast for my kids, of course). And the silence . . . well it is just a wish at the moment! LOL. But I still love that the first thing I do in the morning is something I enjoy. Find something that you can look forward to when you lie down at night, even the simplest thing like mine – COFFEEEEE!

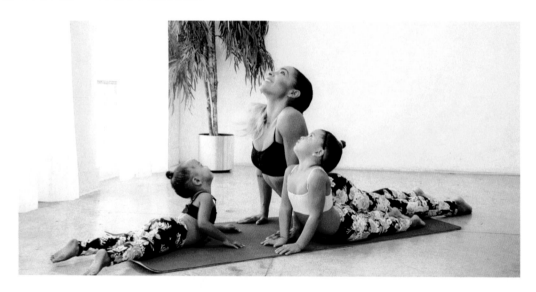

Maybe taking a nice, hot shower or listening to your favorite music or reading the news is what you enjoy. Whatever you do, try to stay away from the gossip sites, because they are so distracting! Social media in general, especially first thing in the morning, should be controlled. I have a rule that I don't check my pages til after I've taken care of getting my kids dressed and fed. I give myself about an hour before I start checking my phone, emails and updates in the morning. Even if that means you have to get up earlier, take a moment without distractions in the A.M! It really does something to your day.

Another ritual I have is drinking a glass of water before anything else goes into my mouth, especially since I am a coffee drinker. I make sure that a glass of water enters my system first thing in the morning and the last thing I drink at night before bed EVERY SINGLE DAY! I also try to drink as much water throughout the day as I can, especially whenever I eat. Also, if you are trying to lose weight, make sure you drink a glass of water before every meal! It is guaranteed to make you eat less. Yes, maybe just a little bit less, but imagine eating less each time you eat. The little bits add up! And what do I always say? A little goes a long way!

I don't take vitamins or anything of that sort, because I make sure that I take in enough fruits and veggies, and foods that give me those vitamins in natural form - magnesium, iron, calcium, zinc, Vitamin B, Vitamin D and C - and all that we should consume on a regular basis. It is proven that a lot of supplements, and especially vitamins, are better absorbed in its raw and natural form than as a subverted version (synthetic supplements) inside of a pill. And I think it is just a personal preference of mine, but there is nothing wrong with the right vitamin supplements. Just make sure you know exactly what you

Day 12

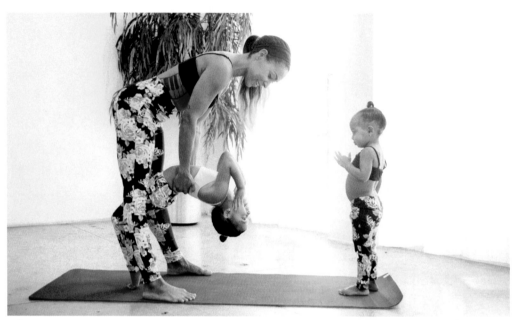

put into your body before swallowing any pills.😉

So, Let's Go! It's our second Yogi Day! Yaay! Remember that YOGA is a journey to find more awareness within yourself and connect to yourself. As you continue to practice, you will understand your body more and adjust accordingly. If a pose seems too difficult, modify it by using blocks or a rope. As long as you try and do what you can you're doing a great job.

Today we are going to practice the Vinyasa Flow from day 5. You can do this flow every day, by the way! Or just get into a posture you feel like your body needs at any given moment. I do just that — like going into a squat when in a long line at the mall or just stretching up in mountain pose while talking to a friend. The awareness you gain by doing yoga is such an amazing thing and that, as well as most other things in yoga, is something that happens with time! So, if you don't feel much at first and aren't sure whether or not you're doing yoga right, just try to focus on feeling the parts of the body that you're using. Another very important thing that is probably the most important when doing yoga is this: DO NOT EVER hold your breath! New yogis tend to hold their breath while in a difficult pose without even realizing it. Be mindful of this and be mindful of your facial expression too. Even if you are struggling in a pose, don't show it. Try to do it effortlessly. In Bikram Yoga the dialogue even has smiling, happy face in it, which encourages you to smile throughout class.

Yes, certain yoga poses require strength that you may have to build up over time, but most poses require stability, and it is easy to get those two confused. Stability may be something you learn by using your strength, but as one of my favorite yogi teachers Dylan Werner says: "Stability is strength without effort." Try to practice techniques without thinking too much about it. I know it's a lot to remember, but this is why we will be doing the same flow throughout the 30 days. You may add on by holding poses longer or changing up the order of poses, which will help guide you into a state of where you **ARE** yoga. ☺

Day 12

Quinoa Salad

My older sister, Sophie, who has been a Vegetarian for many years now, got me into LOVING Quinoa. I never even thought of cooking it, let alone let it be a full meal salad, until she made it for me once in Germany. I never even knew what Quinoa was (shameful). If you're like I used to be, just not aware of what it is, or why you should include it into your diet, here are some facts: Quinoa is considered a "Health Food" because it is a plant-food which is gluten free and high in protein. It is a grain that is higher in fiber than most other grains. It also contains iron, potassium, calcium and Vitamin E, among other nutritious antioxidants. Besides that, it promotes metabolic health! Nothing but good stuff comes from eating Quinoa and best of all, it is delicious! Especially prepared like this

Prep:10 min, Cook: 15 min, Total time:15 min

Prepare

1. In a pot bring 2 cups of water and the quinoa to a boil and immediately set the heat to LOW. (cook for 15min)
2. Cut up all the ingredients into small pieces and prepare the dressing (see recipe from day 2).
3. Place quinoa into a bowl and cool for 2-5min
4. add all of the toppings, add dressing and salt and pepper, ENJOY!

What You Need
(For 2 servings)

1 ½ cup of Quinoa (uncooked)
1 Tomato
¼ cucumber or 2 persian cucumbers
½ cup of olives (any kind you like)
½ Red Pepper
2 oz. feta cheese
salt and pepper

House Dressing (Recipe From Day 2)

FOOD OF THE DAY

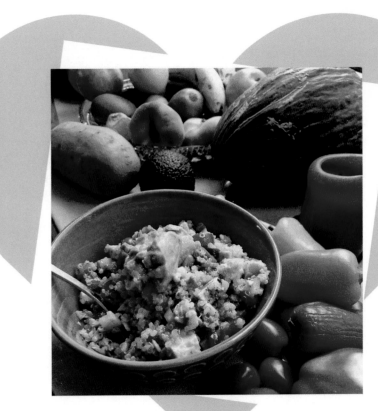

Day 12

Day 13

Heavy Lifting

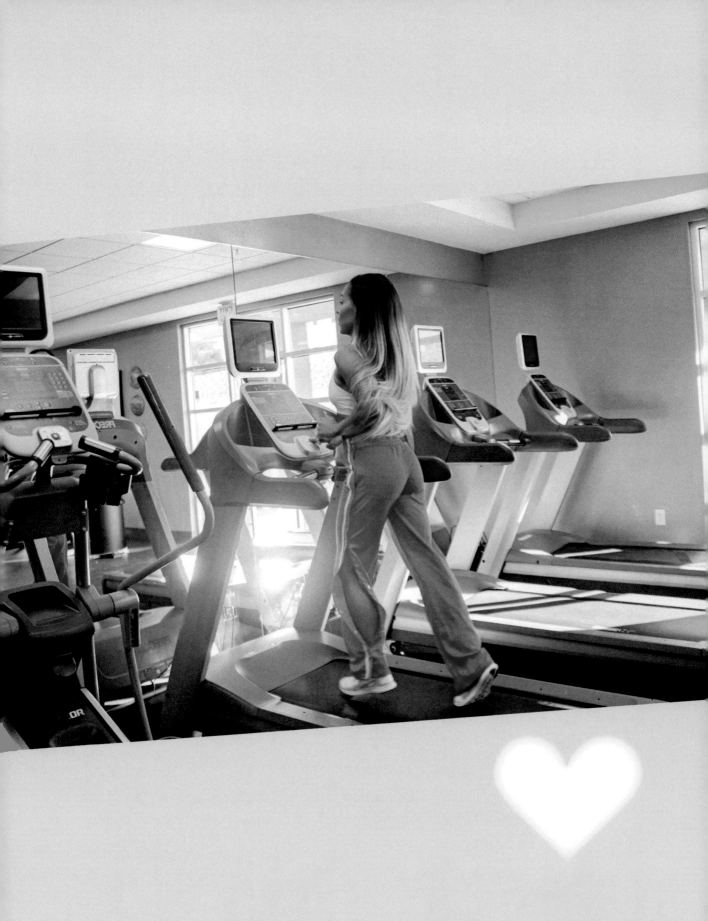

Whatever day of the week it is, I decided to make this day about strength. We all want to be STRONG. We want to be strong both physically and mentally. It has become more of a trend to be strong and fit than anything, it seems. Not that we have to follow trends, but again, it's all about feeling good!

Think about it: If everything in your life felt good, you'd be HAPPY. Happiness depends 100 percent on how you feel — not on what a situation may or may not be or what you have or don't have. Yes, you may feel bad due to a certain event happening in your life or because you can't have something you really want or possibly feel you need, but if that's the case, it is only because you have gotten attached to something outside of yourself. I'm not saying to avoid attachments, but know that with too much of an attachment to things or people, we can lose ourselves easily. Happiness is a choice.

Knowing how amazing it feels to be both fit and strong, especially when I used to be none of the above, I encourage you to work towards "The Fit Life!" As this is YOUR body, you have to live in every day, you should feel good in it and you already are doing big things by getting this book and following my leads! Hooray!

I oftentimes get asked by women, where I get my strength from. Honestly, I built it up from nothing. I used to be the opposite of strong and confident, and I touched on this in my previous book, "The Other

Woman," which is a memoir about my life and experiences with love in the public eye. You can get it on Amazon.com or Barnesandnoble.com. It is amazing to look back and think of the person I used to be. I literally thought I could never be who I have evolved to becoming now. I'm comfortable in my body and with myself — literally fearless and optimistic about the future. And most importantly, I'm STRONG.

I tell women all the time that it was necessary for me to suffer and hurt and feel that pain I felt to gain strength. You can't become strong without conquering a battle and making it through a storm by fighting and falling. People telling you "No" when you believe in yourself is a force of motivation for me — always. Things like that are the very things that make you strong. So even though I sound crazy to people who have watched me go through what I have been through on television, I appreciate the journey and I don't regret anything. Those experiences made me who I am. Those hard times made me STRONG. The moment I packed up and left New York (pregnant with a one-year-old), I only felt strong enough to take that leap because of what happened prior (read "The Other Woman" for more details). Because of how much I had been down, if none of that drama had happened, I would have not had the courage and strength to get up and leave, just like that!

Day 13

*"**Strength doesn't come from what you can do, Strength comes from overcoming the things you once thought you couldn't.**" – Rikki Rogers*

Enough about me, this is about you and your day! I am probably somewhere right now doing the same thing you'll be doing – Heavy Lifting.

This simply means that we are not running, jumping or doing any sort of cardio today. We will directly focus on certain muscle groups. I randomly choose gluteus and lower body! Let's GO!

Exercise:

Do every exercise for 15-20 reps! Then repeat the entire exercise twice. You can do this anywhere from your living room to the park! No weights are needed.

1. Side Lunges:

Start in standing position with your legs together. Step out to the right (a wide step about 3 feet), then bend your right knee and push your butt backwards. Push up to standing and repeat on other side. Do this 15-20 times.

2. Lunge walks (15 steps):

Start in standing position. Step forward with the right leg while keeping the upper body lifted and straight, back knee comes close to the floor, then step up the front foot. Move on with the other side.

3. In-Out Squats:

Start in standing position with feet together. Bend your knees, but don't let them come too far forward. Push your butt back! Come back up, open your legs about 2 feet wide and do the same movement immediately. Repeat! (You can add a jump to make it more intense in-between squats.)

4. Kickbacks:

Start on all fours with knees under chest, hands under shoulders. Come down to your forearms and extend the right leg high up to the sky then bring it back down. Keep moving the same leg up and down for 20 reps then switch to the other leg.

5. Step-Ups:

Find a higher surface, like a bench or a chair. Place your right leg on the chair and step up, then step back down. Switch to the left and keep going back and forth 20 times.

Day 13

6. Hip Bridge:

Lie on your back with knees bent and feet on the floor (not too far out, but rather close to your butt). Lift your butt and squeeze your gluteus until you have a straight line from neck to knees. Come back down to the floor and keep moving up and down. To go a little harder, straighten one leg, point it up to the sky and push your butt up in the same way only the bottom leg.

7. Squat Hold!:

Standing position, feet hip distance apart, squat down and hold for 3 sec. come back up and repeat. remember in squat your knees must stay above your ankles and your butt moves backwards!

8. Lunge Jumps:

Step foward into a lunge, then push up with both feet and jump up to switch legs. (Remember to always bring the back knee as close to the floor as possible while the upper body stays straight.)

MI Spinach Salad

Although spinach isn't my favorite kind of lettuce for a salad, this combo is the bomb!! It's super easy to make and although it makes a great appetizer salad, I will just have a lot of it and make it my main meal, and lunch or dinner is served!

FOOD OF THE DAY

**What You need
(for 3 servings):**

6 oz baby spinach
2oz sliced radish (equals about ½ cup)
½ cup of walnuts (chopped)
½ cup of feta cheese
½ cup of dried cranberries
salt & pepper
My homemade dressing from Day 2!!

Prepare
Mix all ingredients on a bowl, add dressing and toss!

FINISHED

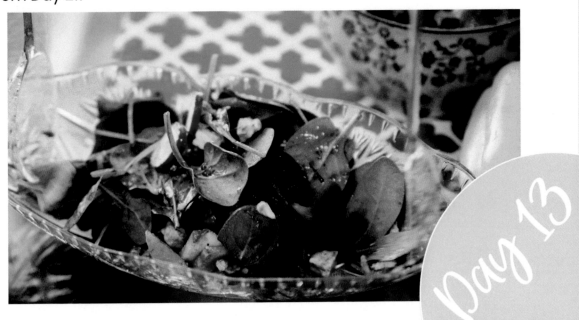

Day 13

Day 14

Walks in The Park

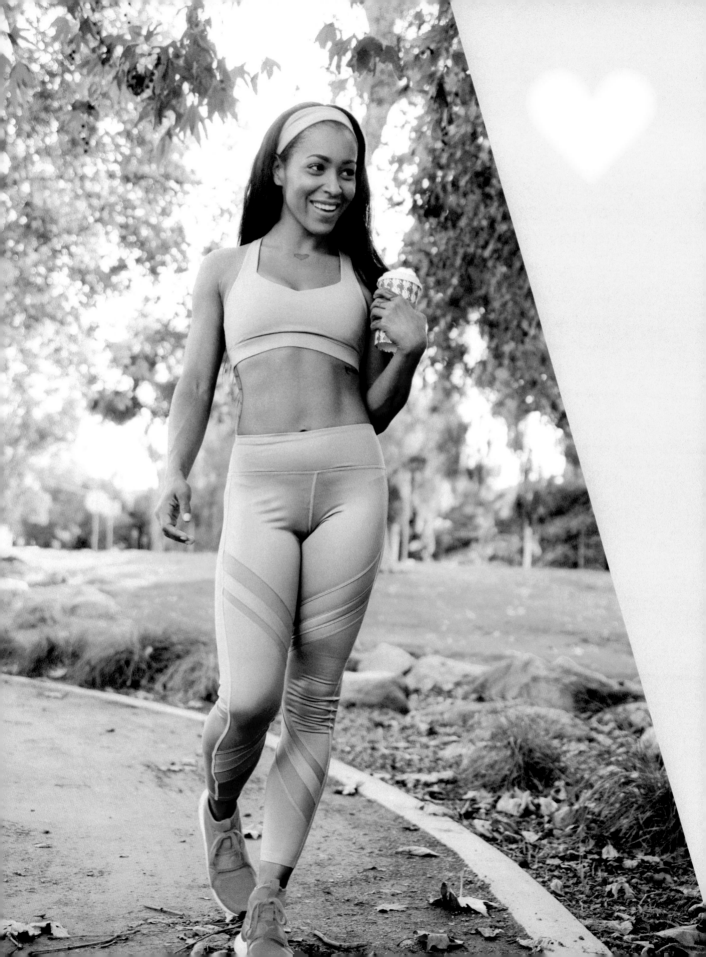

Happy Day 14! You're almost halfway through experiencing life MY way, or at least having a little taste of it in your own life. I hope you're enjoying this journey so far and that the little things I've added to your life have made you feel a positive difference.

A while ago, eight years ago to be exact, I came to the conclusion that "Freedom" is what I need to be happy. Freedom to be myself and do what I want to do. It took me years to figure this out, but ever since I did, I never went back to doing things I didn't feel like I wanted to do, working with people I didn't like because they could possibly 'get me places,' or listening to naysayers or "Faking it til making it." Do you know how many people fake it and never make it? It is just something I have tried, and trying it made me realize I was wasting precious time, because even if I could have "Made It" by faking it longer, it was not worth living unhappy — not a day more than I had. When you live your life knowing there may be no tomorrow is when you can truly live a happy life.

Another important thing is what you do with your free time. When you're a freelance artist and a single mom, like me, time is so limited that it's insane, because every minute you're "free" you want to use that time to work and be creative (at least I do). And at other times you have to take care of the kids, sleep, eat and handle household chores (my laundry literally never stops). When someone asks me, "When are you free?," the true answer is: "Never, but if you're important enough I'll make it happen." That is really what my life is today — busy. It is literally a struggle to fit much else in, but that is when it all boils down to what is important for you and what you enjoy the most. Dating, working out, spending time alone, watching shows, hanging with friends; what do I choose? It's literally about what matters to me the most. I like doing all of the things I named, but I have an order in which they matter to me from most to least, here it is:

Yes, there are way more things you can do for fun and your list may include other things, but these are my top five. What are yours? Of course I left out

1. Working out (I have to make time for).
2. Spending time alone (I also have to make time for, if possible).
3. Hanging with friends and going out (sometimes)
4. Dating (hardly).
5. Watching shows (once or twice a month – LOL).

spending time with my girls, because that's a given! **I always put them first.** They actually can't be on a list, because they are a part of me.

Write your list down below in the order of which matters most important and least important.

_____

_____

_____

_____

_____

_____

_____

_____

_____

_____

_____

_____

Living in California, it is easy to want to be outdoors; I get it. And being able to be outdoors more is one big reason I made that move from New York to California. Living in a good climate can be a life-changer, especially if you're not used to it and were raised in a place where the sky is mostly grey, like in Hamburg, Germany. That, alone, is depressing to me, so if you feel that you are unhappy because you live in a place where the sky is mostly grey, then you should work towards changing that. More on that later!

Anyway, take time today to simply enjoy the things that you have!! I wrote a song once with my sisters when we first started recording our album after we had just gotten signed to Def Jam Records back in 2006. The song was called "Make A Change," in which we sang, "Day by day I'm living my life, complain about the things I don't have, I think I'm missing, but I don't see what really matters is right next to me."

Day 14

I want us to focus today on what we have and love! Today and EVERYDAY. If you look at your life and there is absolutely nothing in it that you love or are happy about, well there you have it; Change has to happen. And it won't unless YOU *change* some things. You are already working on it by reading my book. As long as you know YOU are in control of your life and when you stop blaming others, you can successfully move in the right direction.

Yogurt Bowl

The combination of fruit, nuts and yogurt is just one of a kind. If you loved our Yogurt Bowl from Day 2, you may certainly use those ingredients, but maybe you wanna try some new flavors today! And by the way, this doesn't have to be your breakfast. I eat yogurt in the middle of the day sometimes and it keeps me full for a good minute and motivates me to plan a light dinner instead of a heavy one! 😋

Prep:6 min, Cook: 0 min, Total Time: 6 min

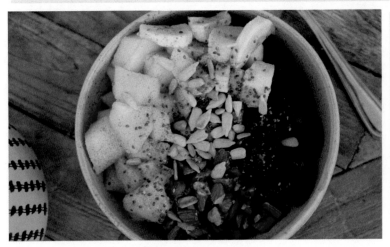

What you need
(for one bowl):

1 ½ cup of low-fat Greek yogurt (plain)
½ banana
½ apple
½ cup of blackberries (or any other berries)
½ cup of almonds (substitute walnuts/hazelnuts/cashews)
1 teaspoon sunflower seeds
1 teaspoon Chia seeds
2 teaspoons honey
½ teaspoon cinnamon

Prepare:
1. Put yogurt in a bowl.
2 .Wash and cut up the apple into small dices.
3. Chop up almonds.
4. Place all of the remaining fruit and nuts into the bowl.
5. Top it with the honey, cinnamon and Chia seeds.

Stir, or eat as is. DONE

Day 14

Day 15

Laugh & Dance

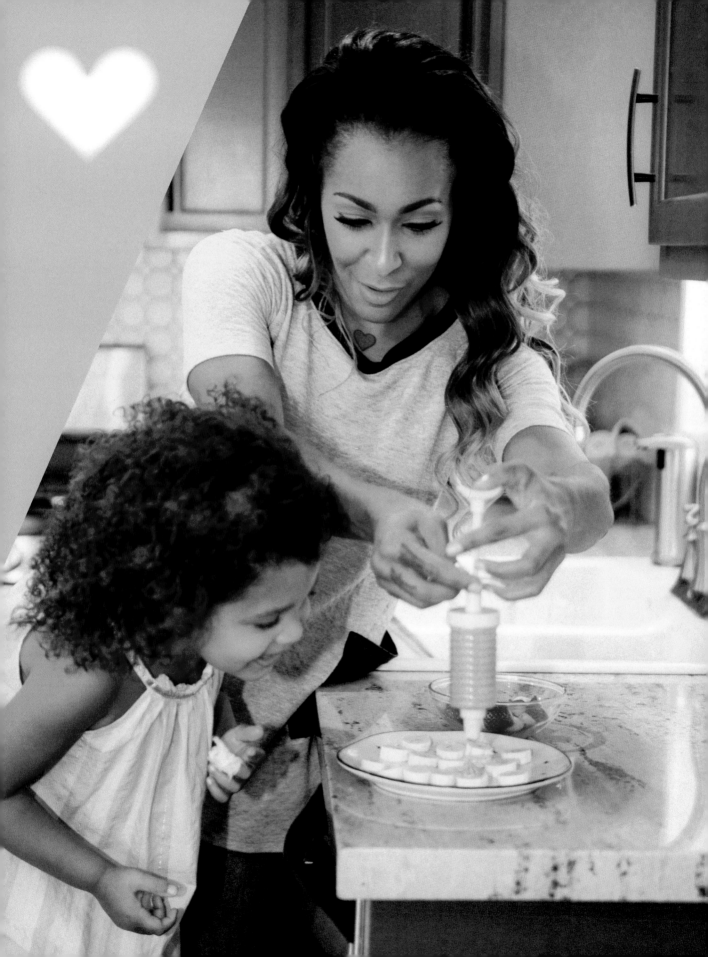

Today I am starting us with a quote that I love by someone unknown.

"STOP OVERTHINKING IT. EAT MODERATELY WELL. WORKOUT A FEW TIMES A WEEK. GET ENOUGH SLEEP. REPEAT FOREVER."

Exactly! All in this quote is the key to a happier life and it is sooooo simple. At least it seems to be. Once you get the hang of it, it'll be easy. In the beginning of anything worthwhile everything you aren't familiar with seems hard, because it is change. Change can even be scary. But it's necessary and it is something you must learn to embrace, especially when you aren't happy.

At one point today, I want you to play music you love. You may be doing this every day already. If so, YAAY, that's great! So many of us get through tough times with music. Music, for me, was literally a lifesaver when I was a teenager. It can completely shift your mood as well.

If you're like me, you'll go to the sentimental, real deep type of songs that make you feel powerful or are simply beautiful. But I have noticed that most people around me get a rush when listening to uptempo, positive music. Yes, I do too. However, I'm a little weirdo who likes different stuff. LOL. Anyway, since my kids have been around, the amount of happy songs we listen and dance to have given me such a new view on what it means to feel a rush of good energy.

Another way of getting a dose of good energy is by surrounding yourself with people who have good energy. Invite a friend over, cook a meal and get some wine (if you like it as much as I do😊). We all know that one person that just always brings us joy. I, luckily,

Day 15

have a couple of those special people in my life. If they're not available, give them a call. I need to take my own advice here. Want to know a little secret? I hate phone calls. But it is good to just interact with someone who can uplift you by simply being there.

Today's goal, and the goal every day is to create a "Happy Space." It's hard for some of us to understand the concept of deciding to be happy. I used to have a hard time getting the grove of it. I used to think, "I can't control how I feel." And truth is, I still can't, but you can learn how to shift your energy towards positivity by simply training your mind to focus on it.

In a recent article in FORBES.com called "How to Be Happy (nearly) All the Time," Jodie Cook explains that no one can hand you a definite formula for happiness, but a definite formula for unhappiness is to worry and stress about things that are completely out of your control. I find that so useful and true, because even though most of us know this, we have to be reminded to not fall into this trap. The worrying and stressing, that is. Jodie continues to say, "Make a list of things that are in your control! Examples: Your attitude, your actions, your words, your thoughts, your choices. Focus on those things and FORGET everything else. Forget things like another's actions, the football score or what people think."

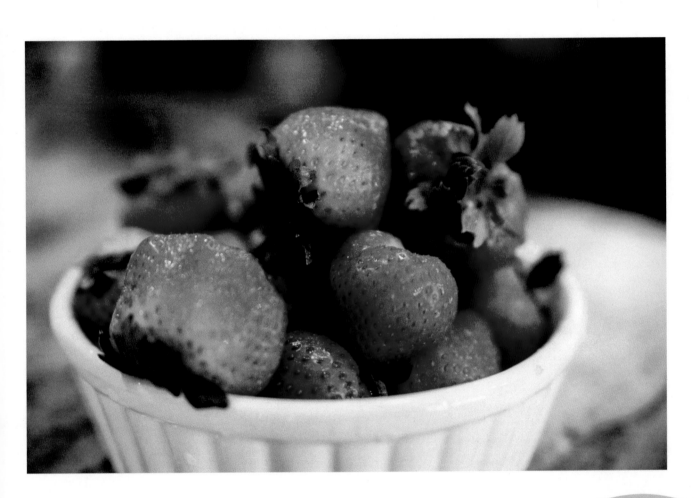

Banana Strawberry Peanut Snack

Less is more! Sometimes even with food! This amazing healthy snack is one of my favorites to have after a workout! I fell for this snack after a famous juice chain discontinued carrying my favorite smoothie, which had peanut butter, banana and berries in it. I would always just dip the banana into peanut butter and have a glass of orange juice along with it. But one day it crossed my mind that all I was missing was the strawberry and I'd have that same smoothie I always loved. And it tastes even better when it's not blended! Again, presenting it as a sandwich makes it just look so super cute and yummy that kids will want to try it! Trust me, my four-year-old wouldn't stop saying "mehr" ("more" in German) after she first had it with me! 😉

Prep: 05 min, Cook: 00 min, Total Time: 05 min

Prepare:

1. Peel the bananas, cut into bite-sized pieces and place on plate.
2. With a spoon, drip a hazelnut-sized amount of peanut butter onto banana.
3. Cut clean strawberries in halves and place one piece onto each banana.
4. Sprinkle with cinnamon.

What You Need (serves 2):

2 bananas
½ pack of fresh strawberries
peanut butter (creamy organic peanuts and salt only, which are my favorite)
cinnamon

DONE!

FOOD OF THE DAY

Day 15

Day 16

Work Harder

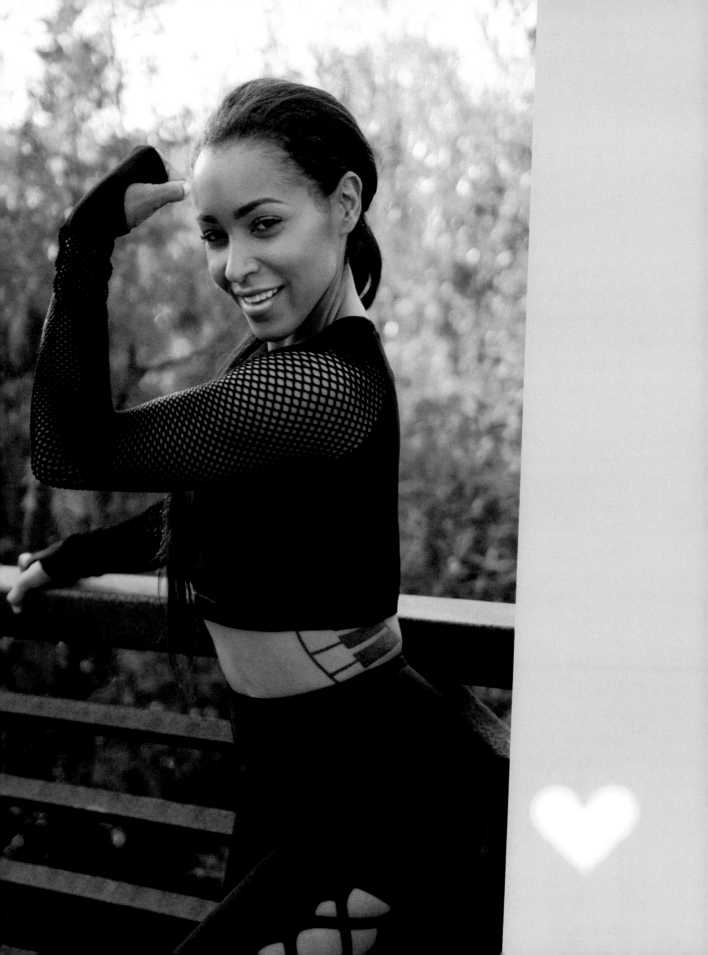

Hello, Gorgeous! If the title of this day doesn't excite you, it's time to change that! I know . . . all these changes right? 😌 But working hard is so rewarding, and you should always be excited about it, even when nobody knows and you work in silence. Thats what I've been doing for years with my music . . . and even now, with this book. At the end of the day, when you work, you get something out of it. Whatever it may be, and whether it will be a success or not, it is YOUR success! Unless you strictly work for the money, you should always work on something you LOVE, and it will eventually bring you money. 😉

Like I said earlier in this book, I get so much joy out of creating a new song, even if it will never become a hit record. I know, for myself, I have created something worthy of making myself and others feel something special. And that alone makes me happy. Personal development makes me happy too. Learning to work primarily on yourself is key to adding value to yourself. Just think what would happen if you made yourself more valuable? Yes, we all want to make more money. Who doesn't want that?! It is a fact that it's not always the one who puts in the most time, but the one who has the most value who wins when it comes down to getting the bread (money). It also puts you in a position to inspire and help more people when you are valued in a professional sense. I must say, your profession has nothing to your personal value. We all have value regardless of stature and money. I learned this from motivational speaker Jim Rohn's seminar on personal development from 1988.

So, whether you work at a job you love or you're an artist doing what you love, like myself, working on yourself and improving your skills in whatever job/ profession you have, is a major key to your own happiness. Now, if you hate your job, then you should put all your energy into your personal development even more. Work on yourself. Work on whatever it is that you want to do every minute you can! Work work, work. And by the way, when you do what you love it shouldn't even feel like work. It may be hard, yes, but it shouldn't feel like work.

An example is when I have to make myself practice the piano because I messed up so much on my last performance (story of my life.) I sometimes don't feel like sitting down and practicing. But at the end of the day, playing keys is a love of mine. I got a whole piano tatted (tattooed) on one side of my body, so why would I ever complain about having to practice? I do have to check myself sometimes though. Yes, it's work, but it's what I want to do. I do want to get better, so there is no way around I've got to work at it.

Day 16

Today's day is called "WORK HARDER" because much like on Day 2, we will work harder than most of the other days! WORK OUT harder, that is! 😌 Are you ready!!??

Option 1:
Take a HIIT Circuit Training Class (If time and money allows).

Option 2:
Take an online (YouTube) 30 minute HIGH INTENSITY workout and finish with 5 stretching poses (of your choice) from Yogi Day.

Option 3:
Repeat FULL BODY excercise from Day 2.

HALLOUMI SALAD
(with homemade dressing)

This recipe was created by my dear sister, Sophie, who introduced me to Halloumi cheese! If you have never had it, don't feel bad. I never even knew what it was before I was in 'Sophie's Kitchen,' about two years ago, and she was grilling it. I didn't understand what was happening. LOL. Grilling cheese? Okay! It looked good and tasted even better! You can get this at pretty much any supermarket. Halloumi cheese is just that, a cheese, so yes, it is pretty high in fat, but it's also high in protein, which makes it a good vegetarian option. I love eating something that is not an animal source food, but gives the same satisfaction. The fact that everything around it is super low in calories makes this a perfectly balanced meal.

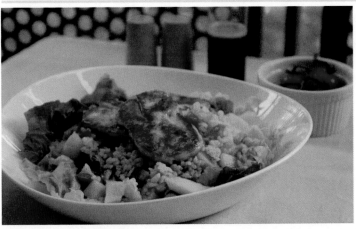

What you need (for 2 servings):
Halloumi cheese (around 8oz)
1 cup cooked quinoa
2 large tomatoes
½ fresh mango
1 lime (squeezed)
lettuce (any kind)
handful of mint leaves
salt & pepper
olive oil
MI salad dressing (recipe from day 2)

1. Mix the cooked quinoa with chopped tomato (tiny pieces), salt, chopped mint and lime juice (half a lime).
2. Chop the lettuce (small) and mix with diced mango.
3. Heat only a little bit of olive oil (1 tablespoon) and fly the halloumi cheese on both sides until crispy (high heat for 1 minute on both sides then lower the heat to medium/low). Cook another 2 minutes (drain any liquid that may build up from the cheese).
4. Serve on a plate, first lettuce/mango mix, then quinoa mix and finally top with dressing and Halloumi cheese! Add salt and pepper to your liking.

Day 16

Day 17

Me, Myself & I

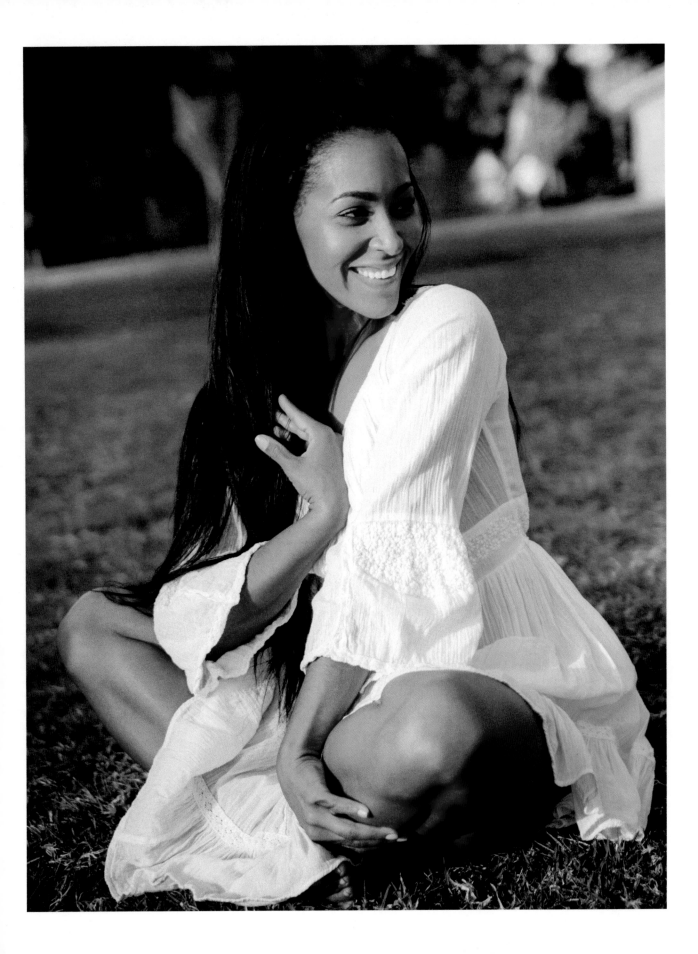

If you're anything like me, you love spending time alone. In my life I have been around and been close to such a variety of different personalities, and it's always been interesting to see how different we all are. Some of us just constantly need to communicate with others, have company and converse, even if it's over text or the phone. I have always been the person who would rather listen than speak. I don't feel like talking much at times and will only speak when asked to in a group setting. That doesn't mean I have nothing to talk about. I just never felt like it was necessary to share. I kept a lot to myself as a teenager, and even now as an adult I still realize I am that loner type person (although I have become a bit more outgoing). It can be a disadvantage when you don't say how you feel at times. It's easy to get misunderstood or simply not be heard. I have had some regrets about NOT saying this or that in some situations and always wondered, "What if I would have," or I've thought, "I should have . . . " But I have learned to accept things I cannot change (for the most part). If it's something that happened in the past or just a few minutes ago, I DON'T STRESS. Instead, I try to do different next time.

Today is all about You. And yes, the fact that you're reading this shows you care about yourself already, and you obviously want to take care of yourself. Yes, our life, and especially as mothers, is definitely not always about us. Speaking for myself, it's mostly about my kids! And I know you'll agree if you're a mom. Chances are you might have a husband or significant other to cater to as well. When that is the case it is easy to let yourself get accustomed to coming last. I have instructed you to take 1-2 hours a day to focus on this challenge with this daily guide, but today I want you to keep YOU in mind, ALL day long! That doesn't mean you're going to neglect your kids, husband, friends and family. It means that in any given situation, you're going to think of yourself.

What would you like to do today? What would you like to eat? What do you want to watch, read or listen to? Yes, someone may get upset, but if they love you, they will get over it in no time!! 😏 If you do have the option of getting some real ALONE time, take it!! You deserve a movie date with yourself, or whatever it is you think you can enjoy solo. I have days where I just go for a drive without having a destination — just to unwind and disconnect from everyone. It's fun for me.

Day 17

FRESH Ginger tea

When I first posted my homemade Ginger Tea on my instagram page @mi_dishes, I had people write me asking which tea used. I found that funny because there is no loose tea or tea bag used here, the fresh ginger combined with boiling water is our tea!! There are many great benefits in drinking this drink especially before bedtime. So have it often — not only today 😊 From boosting your immune system, to helping with digestion and muscle relief, to increasing the blood flow to the brain and hereby energizing it to function at its max, the benefits are endless. Some even say it helps women relieve cramps during their menstrual cycles.

PREP: 1 minute. COOK: 7 minutes TOTAL TIME: 8 minutes

What you need (for 2 cups):
Fresh Raw Ginger Root —
about 3 inches

Prepare:
1. Bring 2 cups of water to a boil in a small pot.
2. While water is heating up first wash, then slice up the ginger root into thin slices. You may also peel it to get all the flavor, but slicing is a pretty good method to get all the juice.
3. Place the ginger into the boiling water and keep boiling on medium-low heat for 7-18 minutes..
DONE!

Add ons:
I drink my ginger tea straight up with no added sweetness but you can totally add some honey or agave and lemon if you like!

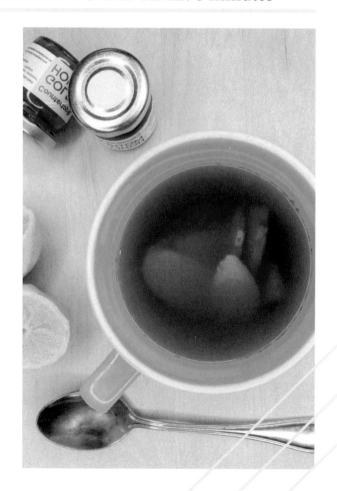

Today's Task:

Make yourself a priority by taking time to do something for YOU. Put yourself first.

Day 17

Day 18

Yogi Day

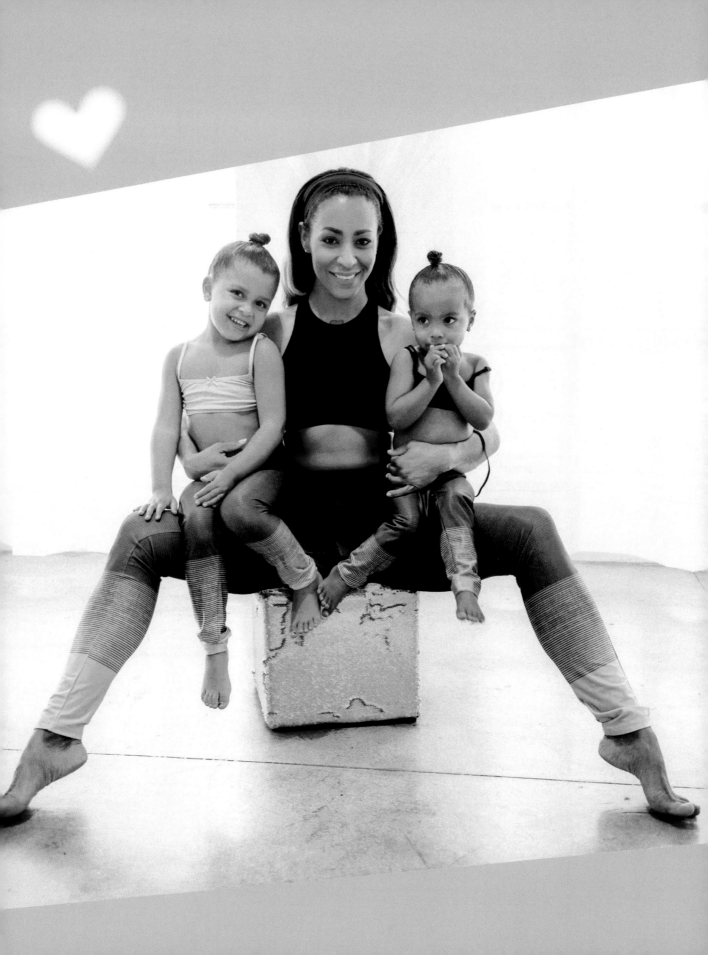

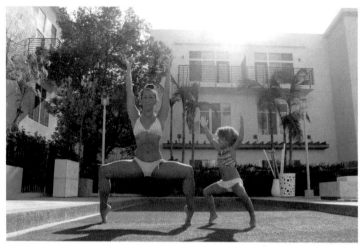

Hey Beautiful! I think that yogi day is my personal favorite because even though I am not a certified yoga instructor, my years of practice have given me this intuitive understanding, and I feel like I just know what I'm doing the most here. In addition to that, it is such a rejuvenating thing to practice. It's such a personal thing. Dealing with a yoga posture can train you to deal better with life events. This has been accurate for me 100 percent. Also, in The Yoga Bible (by Christina Brown), one of the first sentences in the introduction says, "Yoga is being able to relax into who you are," which is a beautiful thing. Read those lines: "Relax into who you are." It feels amazing. No more judging yourself, feeling like you can't do certain things and feeling like you gotta look or behave a certain way. No more feeling the pressure of fitting into society, and no more feeling bad about your flaws or being insecure. All of that, of course, takes time. But I have not felt so comfortable and harmonious in

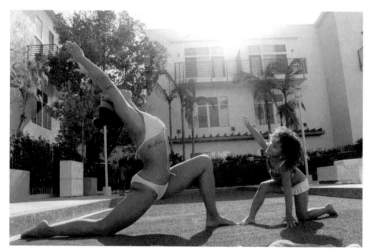

my skin until after I started practicing.

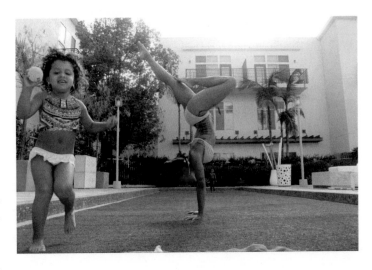

So, yeah, Day 18 is here! We are doing our yoga flow, and if you don't have a quiet moment today, why not try it in the middle of your living room while family life is happening. I know how challenging it is to be in your zone while a toddler screams, "Mommy I gotta go potty" or your teenage kid is nagging you about something (I'm not there yet, whew)! But if you get interrupted, don't worry. An extra challenge is good sometimes. As long as you get through it, no matter when or where, you have done your challenge today! If you do find quiet time or even have the chance to practice outdoors (if the weather is nice), take that time! Connecting with nature while doing yoga is the best, especially in this day and age where all we use all day is electronics and look at computer screens. Get back to the roots for a moment at the park or the beach — or even your own backyard.

Sleep

Another thing I want you to do today is to go to bed early. Making sure you are getting a good night's rest plays such a huge part in your health and happiness. Yes, you can be "Team No Sleep" at times when you have a certain project to finish or really want to get something done by a deadline, but do not make it a habit to not sleep. A healthy body and mind (especially a hard working one) needs rest! Try to even have a sleep schedule where you go to bed and wake up around the same time everyday! There are many benefits here! I have read on many different science blogs and articles that having a sleeping pattern has positive effects on your life length, weight loss, focus, skin, immune system, interacting socially and the list goes on.

Some of us are obsessed with looking good because, yes, when you look good, you feel good. But have you ever thought about it in reverse — that when you feel good you look good too? This type of looking good can't be bought! It's a happy glow that only shows when you feel good on the inside. When you take care of yourself. Yes, you can pay to get facials, your hair and makeup done, or even get any type of other treatments and surgeries.

But you can't pay to have that radiance — that inner glow that just makes you more beautiful. This is what I want you to have! And then whatever else you like to do to feel pretty, of course, go ahead. But at the end of the day, it all comes back down to feeling good, which is what I strive for every day of my life, because feeling good equals what? Yes, HAPPINESS.

Tomato Mushroom salad

I once wanted a salad, so I looked into my fridge and discovered I didn't have anything in there for the kind of salad I thought I wanted. All I could find was grape tomatoes corn and an onion. I also had a few mushrooms left, so I said, "Wait a minute! I think I can work with this!" So, I started making this dish, and My kids LOVE it!

FOOD OF THE DAY

Prepare:
1. Chop up the tomatoes and dice the onion.
2. Heat olive oil and sauté sliced mushrooms for about 3 minutes on medium heat (add salt and pepper).
3. Mix everything in a bowl, then add the feta, corn and dressing.
4. Add more salt and pepper and sprinkle with garlic powder.

What you need (for 2 servings):
2 large tomatoes or a pack of grape tomatoes (10 oz)
½ small onion
4 oz white mushrooms
2 tables of feta cheese
½ cup of sweet corn
2 tablespoons of olive oil
garlic powder sprinkle
Homemade dressing (recipe from day 2)

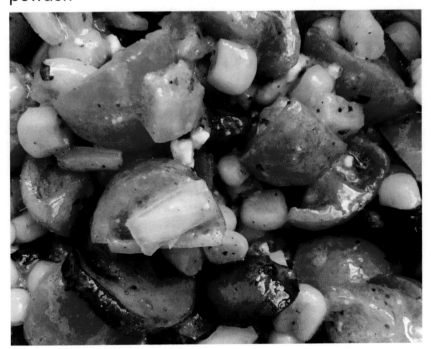

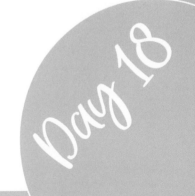

Day 18

Day 19

Park Flow

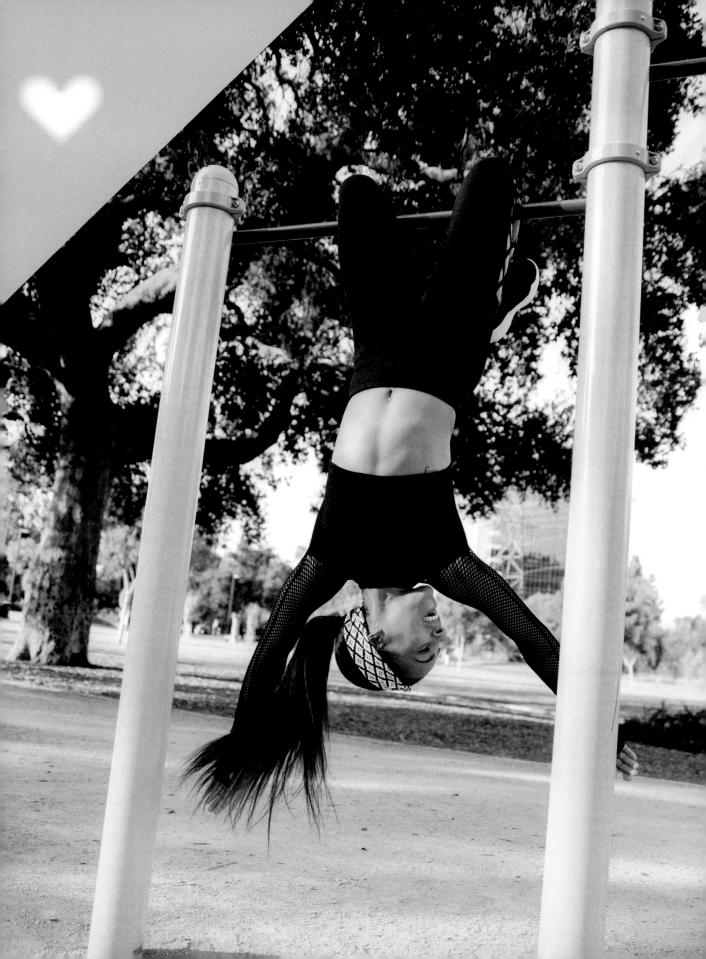

FEARLESS. This is the word I am assigning to you on this day and I randomly picked Fearless today because I had a bunch of de déjà vu moments to-day.. Just FYI, as i'm writing this, it's December 19, 2018 - 11:05pm. Because the year is coming to a close and I am sitting here reflecting all day, moments of my life keep crossing my mind where I recall being brave! Looking back, I even "wowed" myself a few times. From coming to America, to walking out of my record deal into financial crisis, to spending Christmas alone in Hawaii, to moving across the country with a 1-year-old while preggers, to being honest about my mistakes and putting my personal life on national TV for the world to see and judge. There have just been a lot of moments I reminisced upon today. A quote I posted yesterday on my social media (actually one of my favorite quotes) says **"SHE WHO IS BRAVE IS FREE."** This is true, so Take Risks and Jump! Maybe you're nervous and hesitating because something you want could fail big time, but it could also bring a positive outcome. YOU MUST TRY!

I don't know, but even with my sweet, quiet, sort of introverted personality, I really can't think of one thing that I'm afraid of in this life — except something happening to my children or loved ones. But for myself, there is nothing that scares me. Nothing. Yeah, maybe a scary movie or one of those green Chinese beetles flying around here in Cali, or a takeoff on a flight scares me, but these are momentary scares. I'm talking about real fears. I don't have them and that is part of why I can live life so freely.

Ask yourself, what are you scared of? What are your biggest fears?

Write them down below:

_____

_____

_____

_____

_____

_____

_____

Whatever day it is today, insert today's date here:

_____

and mark it as "FEARLESS" day on your calendar. Because from here on out you will work towards erasing those fears! YOU CAN DO IT!

Day 19

I want you to fall into bed tonight (and every night) feeling like, "Today was a good day!" No, you will never have ONLY good days (I have bad days still), but we want to work towards having predominantly good ones! And as well as that, work on looking at and handling the bad days like it's a piece of cake.

Yes, I named today "Park Flow," but you don't necessarily have to go to the park! I want you to do something fun with the kids. I do it so much, and I must admit, my kids are so spoiled that the first thing they ask every morning is, "Mommy, where we going to-day?" LOL. What have I started? Depending on whether or not you're a mom, and also depending on your child's age, find somewhere to go that will be fun for you both. You may say something like, "But my kids don't behave when I take them places," or "We enjoy being home mostly." Well, here's my *Toddler-Mommy* talk for today:

Doing the same things will keep you in the same place. This is the month of change, the month of new activity, even if they are small changes. And here goes my mantra again: A little goes a long way. 😉

Kids follow your footsteps. They learn from you the most, at least when you spend enough time with them. They copy you and want to do what you are doing. They are a mini you and a reflection of you for a reason. You are their example. My kids eat good foods because they see me eat them. They do yoga poses because they see me do them. The best thing to do is let them see you do something good — not just watching TV or looking at something on your phone all the time. Most people do those things when at home.

The entire previous paragraph is pretty ironic, because people used to tell me all the time that I was giving my girls a bad example by letting their dad play me. Yes, I did let that happen, and probably for too long, but what matters is that I always cared about my daughter first. Cori, my now 4-year-old was the only one I had at that time. I made sure I didn't fight in front of her - Ever! I would wait days sometimes to address something, because I had her on my hip non-stop. But of course, kids feel everything. They even feel suppressed sadness. However, once she actually saw me broken down, with tears rolling down my face, I looked at her and her confusion, and that was the moment that made me get out. Read more on that in my first book, "The Other Woman." But what I'm saying is that what matters is that you eventually show your kids that strength, confidence, happiness and self care is so important. Even if you have to build those things up from nothing, start — step by step. Most of us know this, yet we get caught up in situations where we feel helpless.

Day 19

The only way out of helplessness is TAKING CON-TROL. It starts with awareness and knowing your worth. When I first started putting out music independently and without a record label, I went through a phase of praising the phrase : "I AM." As a result I named my first ever solo EP just that. The second project, I named "I AM: Part 2." And I even went as far as getting it tat-tooed on my fingers. " I AM," without anything behind it, because they are just such powerful words stand-ing alone. To me it has always been an expression of self awareness. I AM worthy, I AM somebody, I AM amazing, I AM whatever the hell I wanna be! Because for years, in my professional life, all I had heard was all of the things that I was NOT. I gained my confi-dence back by remembering that actually I AM a lot of things they either missed or ignored for selfish, egoistical and greedy reasons. Whatever I wasn't, just wasn't meant to be.

In 2011 I wrote something that I want to share here, because I recently stumbled upon it and I thought it was just interesting to see how the whole "I AM" thing started:

I always wanted...but NOW...

I always wanted to be a great singer, now I wanna be a great musician

I always wanted to become famous, now I want
to become happy

I always wanted to have lots of money, now I
want lots of love

I always wanted recognition, now I want respect

I always wanted to be the best, now I want to
be MY best

I always wanted to convince them, now I need
them to convince ME

I always wanted to be heard, now I want to be
understood

I always wanted to impress others, now I wanna
impress myself

I always wanted to change me, now I wanna
change the world

I always wanted to be somebody, now I AM

German Rice Pudding

(Milchreis)

I literally grew up on this! In Germany we have a specific type of rice which would be similar to short grain rice. However, it is possible to achieve the creamy texture with long grain rice, which is more common in America, as long as it's cooked longer! This is best with whole milk, but if you're trying to save calories go with low-fat milk. I always do it and it tastes great to me!! The cherries are a must! So, go find a Trader Joe's or order some dark morello cherries on Amazon! It is, to me, what makes the dish! Enjoy.

Prepare:

1. In a large pot, bring the milk to a boil. Add the rice and immediately turn the heat to LOW.
2. Add sugar and vanilla, then stir.
3. Cook for 45 minutes on low heat, stirring every few minutes (if consistency is too thick, add more milk). You wanna achieve a yogurt thickness for this dish.
4. Add one egg yolk and stir thoroughly.
5. Serve hot in a bowl, sprinkle more sugar and cinnamon and top it with the cherries.

This can, of course, also be eaten cold!

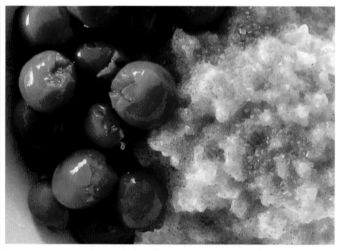

What you need (for 4 servings):
1 cup of long grain white rice
6 cups of milk (your choice)
3 tablespoons of brown sugar
cinnamon
1 egg yolk
1 teaspoon of vanilla extract
Dark Morello cherries

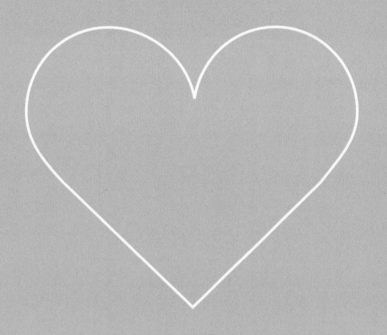

Day 20

Sweat!

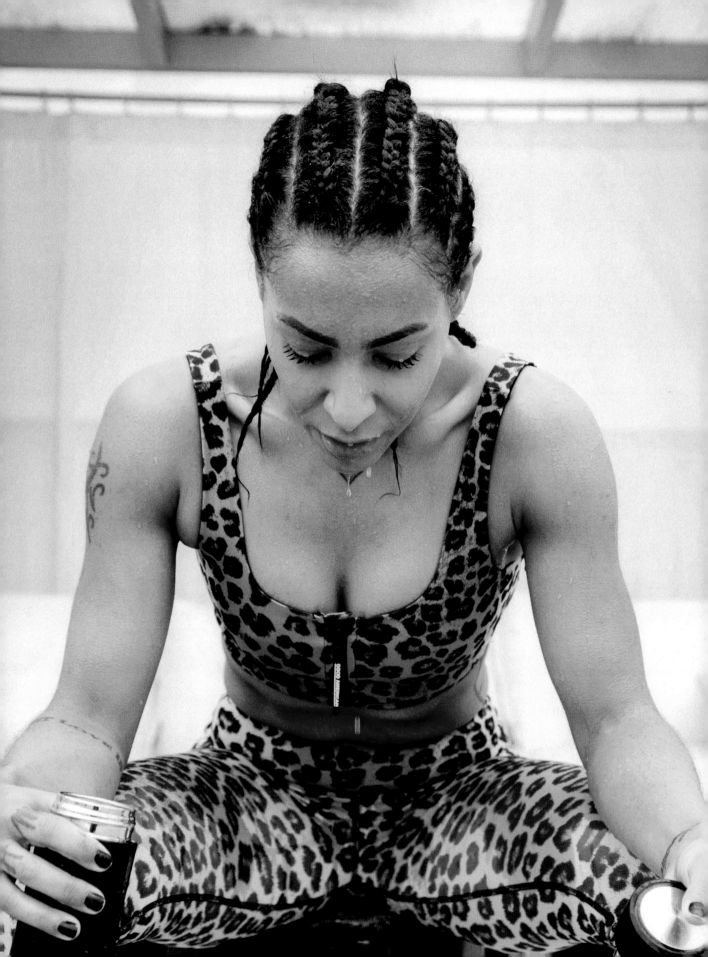

Hi, Queen! Hope you had a bomb day yesterday and a good night's rest, because the intensity of today's workout is HIGH! We need to make sure after a few days of light (or no workout) we completely exhaust ourselves. I also hope that you keep track of your food intake! Or should I say, Be Mindful. I definitely don't write down what I eat or anything like that! No counting calories because I feel it messes with the mind. Yes, I'm giving you recipes of things I normally eat, but obviously you're still adding on to them, as I am not giving you a   complete nutrition guide here. Just think about what you had yesterday when preparing for the new day. If you ate pretty healthy yesterday, it's okay to have a little more today, especially when you work hard!! If you had dessert yesterday, pass on it today though. We just want to get rid of the idea of having to DIET! It literally ruined me as a teenager! I suffered from all sorts of eating disorders even anorexia for a year, and the thoughts I had about food used to make me feel Ill. We don't want to have anxiety about what to eat, feel restricted, think of numbers, a scale, following rules and

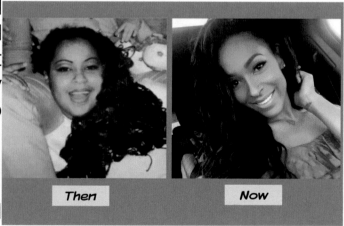

Then   Now

such things. We want to be at ease. We want to feel excited about eating, and be calm when we do, and happy, eating with peace of mind and enjoyment! In my personal journey, I used to feel all of the anxiety of the first things I mentioned, but now, I feel all the last ones I mentioned, and it seemed so impossible at first. I thought I could never become happy in my body. But here I AM . . . okay with my imperfections and learning to love them.

For today I suggest mixing cardio and weights/ strength exercises. Just like in all of our PINK days we need an hour of sweating!!

My go-to is always the treadmill or running outdoors, but as I noted before, jumping rope continuously for 30 minutes (2 minutes on, 2 minutes off) has been an amazing switch-up for me! And I savor the moments when my kids are with me, because I can keep an eye on them at all times while sweating.

On today's HIGH-Intensity day, a great thing to do (as always, we're getting into the routine) is to also take a HITT class! Choose one of the workouts from Day 2 today, and we are in business!

Day 20

Jalapeño pizza from scratch

Who doesn't love pizza!? Even though there are so many amazing pizza places around, try making this from scratch on a fun day like today where you definitely deserve it! This pizza is meatless and limited in toppings but less is more here! It also is a great way to bring family (espicially kids) together and have quality cooking time. You can also add additional toppings to your liking! And/or Add any of the salads in this book as a side dish. It always makes a better meal when you add your greens. ☺ Enjoy.

Prep: 10 min, Cook: 5 min, Total Time: 15 min

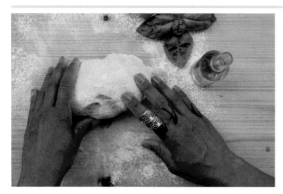

What you need
(for 3 Pies):
0.2 oz dry yeast (equals about 1 ½ teaspoons)
4 cups of flour
2 tablespoons of olive oil
1 ½ teaspoons of salt
1 ½ teaspoons of sugar
1 cup of warm water

For the topping:
1 glass (24oz) marinara sauce
2 8oz bags of shredded cheese (sharp or mild cheddar)
1 12oz jar of jalapeños

Prepare.
1. Mix all the ingredients into a large bowl (yeast and water last).
2. Keep mixing with a dough hook (or your hands if you don't have one) for 8 minutes.
3. Cover the dough with a kitchen towel and let it sit for 30 min in a warm space (you can use your oven for this, just set it to 125 but make sure you turn it OFF completely once temperature is reached, then place the bowl with the dough inside, and just let it sit in there for 30min).
4. Take the dough out of the bowl and kneed it with your hands for another good 5-8 minuses.
5. Separate the dough into 2-3 pieces and spread it out with a rolling pin, then add marinara sauce, jalapeños and cheese.
6. Place it into the oven at 425 degrees for about 10 minutes until the dough looks crispy and cheese golden!

FOOD OF THE DAY

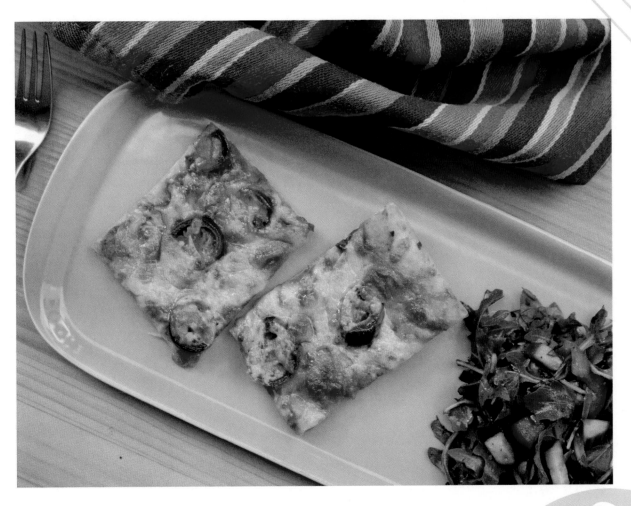

Day 20

Day 21

Pamper Yourself

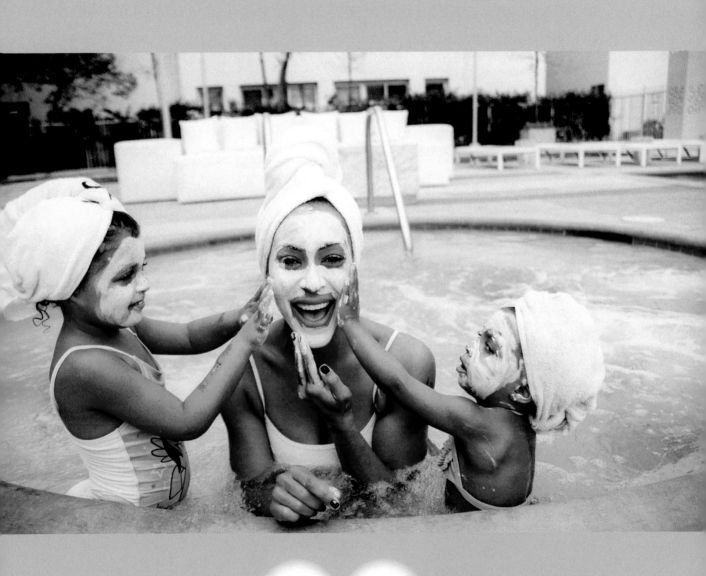

Happy 3 weeks, Beautiful!!! Here's to another FUN day! Whatever your schedule is today and whatever you have to take care of on your "To Do" list, and whatever your job requirements are, take 2 hours to do 2 things:

1. BUY YOURSELF SOMETHING!

In my life these days I find myself stuck between needing to save money or telling myself, "You only live once." However, if I keep things balanced, everything always works out — just like in anything else that we do. I used to always be overly responsible and pass on things I wanted because I was only thinking about the future. But in the past few years I've done more of "You only live once," and it's done good for my happiness. I know a lot of people, even in my close circle,

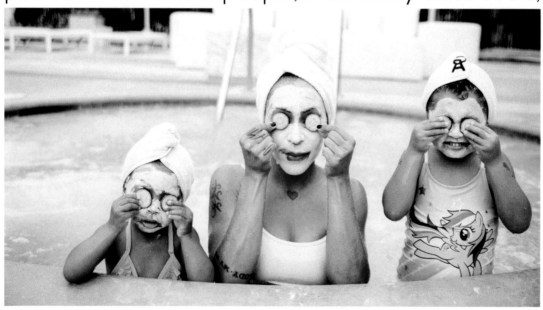

that always have the "You only live once" mentality. Although that may sound about right, knowing when to say, "No" and knowing when to say, "Yes" is so important (and not just when it comes to your pockets). Make a habit of doing things in moderation, but repeatedly. I'm not a financial adviser, but I'm here to share my experiences in life and the things that have changed my life for the better. Not giving a crap sometimes feels good though. 😏

Plus, you deserve good things, and shopping can lift your mood! Get yourself something you've been wanting to have, but haven't gotten it because you think you just can't spend the money right now. Many of us might not buy for ourselves because we buy so much for our kids (me, all day)!! I hardly shop for myself anymore, but that is why it's so much more special whenever I do. We all don't have money to just shop at any given moment (and I've definitely been there), so if you're too broke to buy something, go window shopping and note three things you would LOVE to have! Work towards it! 😊 Make sure you put some makeup on and dress cute and walk through the mall feeling like you deserve everything you see. Besides, the mall is always a nice walk. And walking is what? Yes, excercise!

Day 21

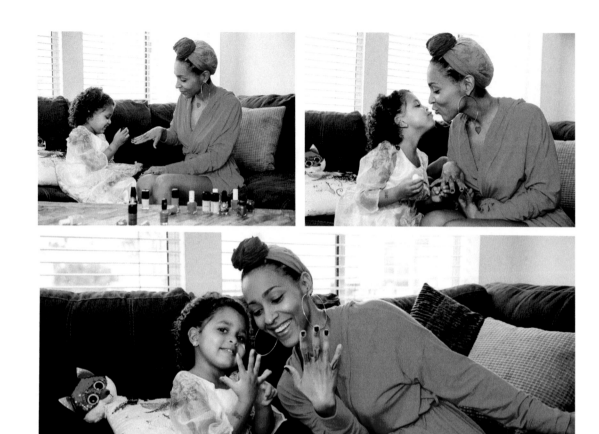

2. HIT THE SPA!

It always feels good to get a fresh mani and pedi … or even a massage. But, again, if money is an issue, simply make your own "spa at home" day! My kids and I do it all the time! It ain't hard! Put on a detoxifying mask, and watch your favorite show while your bath is pouring, then Relax. You may have to wait for the bath until your kids are asleep, which in my house, is more relaxing because I won't hear, "Mommy are you done?" every three minutes. LOL.

Make your house smell nice by using scented

candles or oils, and put on some jazz music. If you're not into jazz, maybe some R&B slow jams will do it for you. And you can always listen to some of my songs. 😉 Just create a relaxing atmosphere where you can zone out for a minute. If you've never done your nails before, why 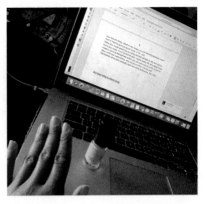 not give it a try? Actually, I'm giving myself a mani right now, while I'm writing this book — NO LIE!

A lot of people, especially women these days, thrive on having money to get everything done and even like to brag about it on social media. I, on the other hand, thrive on doing things myself (even when I do have the money to get it done)! I love it! I feel a sense of accomplishment and power when I do something that others pay lots of money for. Even my body is part of my own doing. Self-made, Baby!

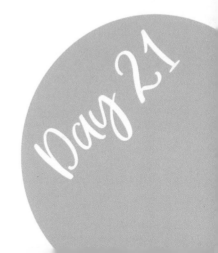

Day 21

Celery Soup

(Blender Required)

Healthy is my way to go on days I don't work out! At least, I try. This recipe comes from my beloved mom who is going to kill me for substituting heavy cream with coconut milk! OOPS. However, I tried both versions, and it is still as yummy as ever without the cream! Try substituting the coconut milk with cream if you like, but if you're trying to be healthy today, cook it with the ingredients I listed! You can also skip the bread. I won't, but hey, some of us may really be out to lose some inches, so skipping bread whenever you can might be your choice. ☺ My personal tip: Use lots of chili for the spicy effect! YUM!

Prep:07min Cook:23min Total Time:30min

Prepare:
1. Peel celery and cut in 1-inch cubes.
2. Cut onion and ingwer into small cubes as well
3. Peel and cube uncooked potatoes
4. Heat Olive oil into pot
5. Sautee ingredients for 6-8 minutes, medium heat until golden brown while stirring.
6. Add sugar.
7. Add water.
8. Add salt & pepper.
9. Boil on moderate heat for 15-20 minutes.
10. Place into blender and blend until even.
11. Add coconut milk.
12. Stir with a whisk.
13. Sprinkle nutmeg.
14. Sprinkle chili (if you like spicy).
15. Chop fresh parsley and sprinkle on top.

Ingredients (for 2 servings):
1 celery root
1 large onion
3 inches fresh ginger (about 1 ounce)
3 Med sized Potatoes
½ cup of coconut milk
2 cups of water

Seasonings:
salt & pepper
parsley
nutmeg
1 tablespoon brown sugar
chili

DONE!

FOOD OF THE DAY

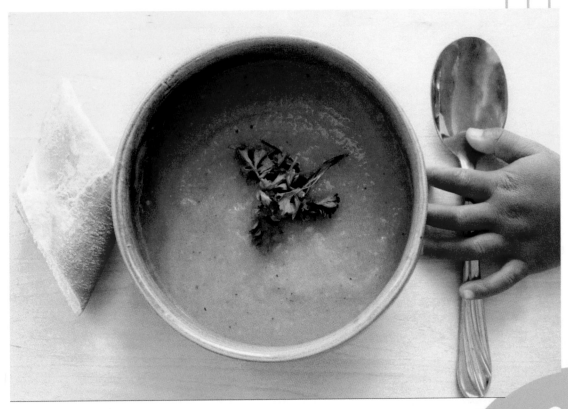

Day 21

Day 22

Explore A New Place

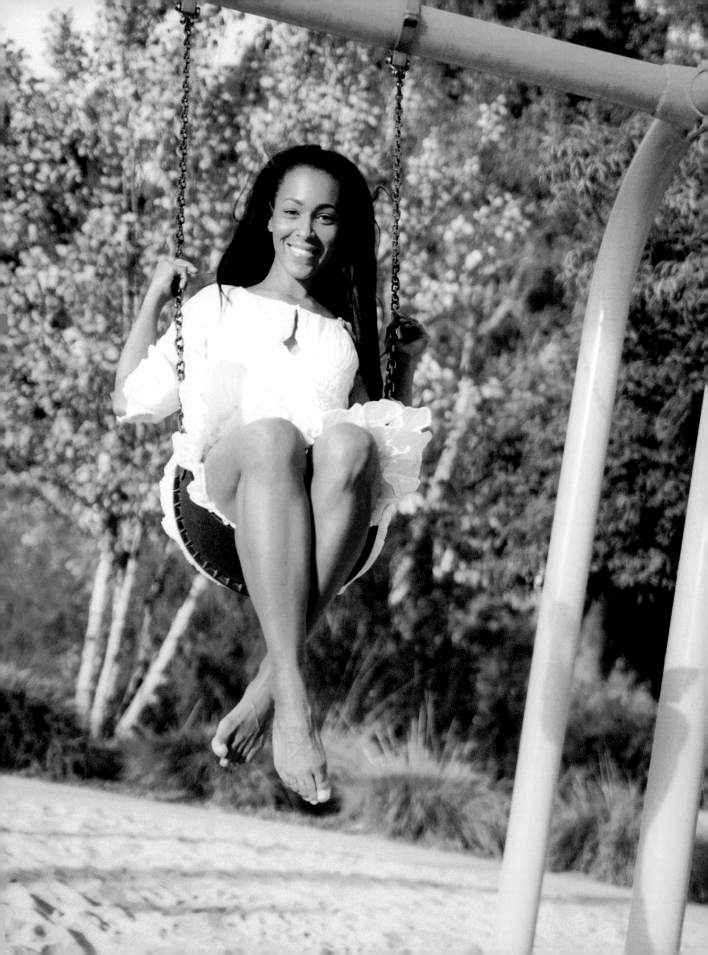

So ... it's Day 22. I hope you're still with me at three weeks in, and honestly, I hope this feels fun, as it does for me. Today and everyday, (but especially today) is about Enjoyment. Having a routined life is a good thing to a certain degree, but when you don't see, feel, hear, smell new things, it's hard to get new inspiration and easy to get bored without realizing it. Maybe you just feel blah. And it could be because you are missing excitement! And by excitement I don't mean anything major like a vacay or helicopter ride. It could be something as simple as visiting a cute store you've never visited or taking the train instead of driving. It's the little things! You may think you're happiest in your comfort zone, or you may love being home (like me), but to be fully happy you must be adventurous. At least that's what I believe!

"Fill your life with experiences, not things. Have stories to tell, not stuff to show." anonymous

I often find myself having a hard time making decisions about whether I should do something or not do it. I recently started to tell myself to ALWAYS go with DOING it! Just GO! Whatever it may be, because in life we are more likely to regret the things we didn't do than the things we did.

I love taking walks in new surroundings! Since I had my kids I've developed a passion for finding new playgrounds, parks or places for them to have fun! But even for myself; I love going somewhere new, like a new bar or a new area in town that I haven't explored. Get out, even without having a specific place to go. With me being a coffee fanatic, I always end up at some new coffee spot and I can't tell you how much that excites me!

A little story: When I spent a week alone in Kauai, Hawaii in December of 2013, I was on this beautiful resort that had everything to offer and most people who stayed there spent all their time in the restaurants, by the pool, on the beach or on one of the many tours the resort had to offer. But I rented a car and drove, without a map (Yes, I had my phone and google map in case of emergency), but without having a destination in mind, I ended up in a place so beautiful that I couldn't remember to take a picture of it. I will forever remember the view from a mountain-top with trees so pretty and the amazing smell of the ocean, and the tropical breeze with a horizon so gorgeous that it literally took my breath away.

Day 22

Those are the moments and memories that make life amazing. Yes, I could have been scared all by myself with no one else around around, but I wasn't because I felt happy there while going through such a rough time in my life.

Have you ever noticed that the happiest people are adventurous, active, traveling and don't dwell on materialistic stuff much? They are the ones who go out and see new things, the people who are spontaneous and not afraid of something challenging. Those people really LIVE life and don't just exist day-to-day.

Task

Find a place to visit and take a picture of something beautiful there. Put the photo in a folder in your phone called (NEW PLACES). See, where i'm going with this is beyond this book, because every month you should add to your folder to eventually have a collection of NEW PLACES. Photos you can show! Or you can just keep the photos for yourself and look at them to remember that specific day you did something new. Cute idea, right? I have just recently started this myself and it is FUN!

Ohhh how I wish I had that picture from my Kauai story!!

Grilled Chicken & Onion Salad

Follow the recipe from Day 2: Simple salad with homemade dressing, instead of Romain, maybe you'll want to try a different Green Leaf Lettuce, or a spring mix, just to switch it up! You can also substitute the Dill Pickle for Bread and butter pickle which has a sweet taste and is MY personal fav with chicken salad!

Prep:15 min, Cook: 5 min, Total Time: 20 min

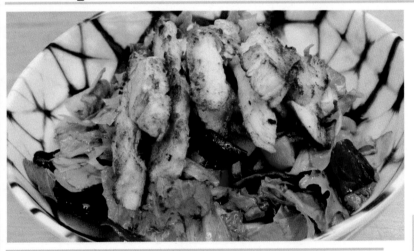

What You need (for the chicken):
1 chicken breast (4-6oz)
olive oil
seasoned salt
garlic powder
pepper

Tip: You can cut the chicken raw before cooking it and it will be done faster. Cook forjust about 2 minutes

Prepare:

1. Heat oil in a pan.
2. Clean and season the chicken with the seasoned salt, pepper, paprika and garlic powder.
3. Place the chicken in the pan and cook on each side for about 3 minutes, make sure the heat stays on medium to high, and once golden brown, med-low.
4. Season with garlic powder, pepper, seasoned salt while cooking.
5. Slice the chicken into bitesize pieces and top the salad with it!

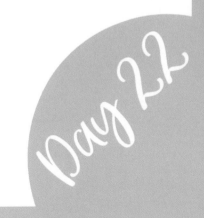
Day 22

Day 23

RUN & Stretch

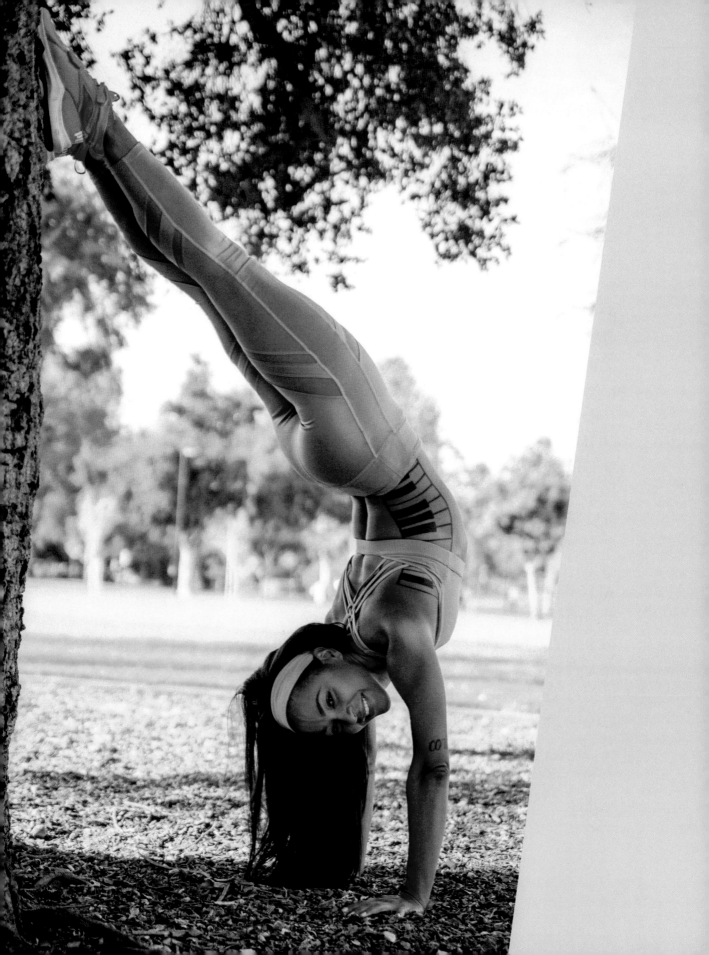

As you can tell, even though we have different days where we do different things, we are also starting to repeat activities and do what we are slowly getting familiar with! However, today our workout consists of two things: We will mix cardio and yoga! MY fav kind of combined workout for the body! For some reason I feel best when I do both of these within one hour. First, we will bring your heart-rate up and get into a sweat!! And I'm talking about a dripping sweat — not just a little steam. 😉 You get the point. I want you to go hard! Today is a PINK day and that means Hard Work!! If you have noticed, there are only a total of 9 PINK days in my 30-Day guide. That is literally how many days a month I go hard on average. People think I work out like crazy every single day. Yes, most days I do *something* for my body, whether it's my walks, my runs, my yoga, my park play with the girls or my resistance and strength training, they're ALL my workouts. Super light or super heavy is irrelevant, as long as I am moving. Only on these 9 PINK days do I really, really GO HARD. Of course that varies from month to month, and I may have 6 PINK days in June, but 13 in July and 8 in August. You get the point though. You don't have to be exact — just get it in.

Repeat the run on the treadmill or outdoors from Day 5. After that, basically just stretch it out like this: Follow Yoga flow from day 5. Pose 1-13! I have noticed that people often skip the stretch, especially in high intensity classes after the workout is done. Many like to leave class right away and skip the stretching, although the after class stretches are already extremely brief most of the time.

Improving your form when exercising, and even when you're not exercising, is a result of stretching. So is reducing stress, preventing injuries, sleeping better and strengthening your muscles. So, I never skip my stretching! I will, at times, just do a quick twist or forward fold and call it a day, but on a day like today we want to make sure we really focus on it as much as we do on our run!

Elsasser Apple Pie

This Dish's Origin is France! But I fell in love with it, again, through my mom. This is my favorite apple pie because it's not super sweet, like most American pies. Less sugar is always a plus. It does contain cream and eggs, so if you're Vegan, this isn't for you. But the special thing about it is that the dough is made with white wine, which gives it that one of a kind taste! You will never want to eat regular apple pie again!

Prep:10 min, Bake: 50 min, Total Time: 1 hour

What You Need:

For the Dough:
2 cups of flour
1 cup soft butter (not melted)
3 tablespoons sugar
½ cup white wine

For the Topping:
5 Apples
3 Eggs
1 Cup of cream
2 Tablespoons of sugar
1 Tablespoon Vanilla exract

Prepare:

1. Mix flour, butter, sugar and wine to a soft mass.
2. Place into greased baking pan.
3. Peel apples, cut in halves and remove seeding.
4. Place apples (round part up) into baking pan (close so that they cover the dough).
5. Put 3 small slices into each apple just so they can absorb the heat properly.
6. Sprinkle the apples with sugar.
7. Pre-heat the oven to 350.
8 .Bake for 30-35 minutes in the middle of rack. When the apples are golden, remove from oven.
9. In a small bowl, put cream and whisk in the eggs, sugar and vanilla extract.
10. Pour mix over the mass and place back into the oven for another 15 minutes, until solid.

Let the pie cool down and ENJOYYYYYY!

FOOD OF THE DAY

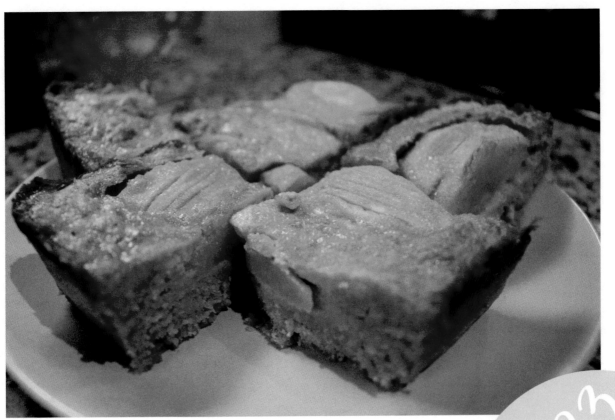

Day 23

Day 24

Lazy Day

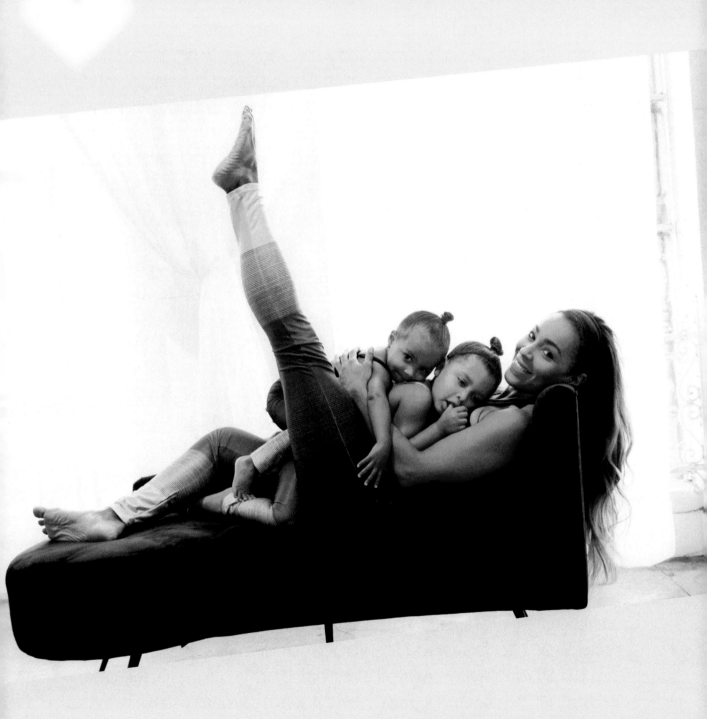

Don't it sound nice?😌 Yes, the best thing is to sometimes be lazy and stay in bed as long as you'd like!! Maybe you're one of those people who don't have an early job or babies that wake up early in the mornings. If so, enjoy, because even on my "Lazy days" I have to get up and get going in the mornings. It's good to take that extra hour of rest if you can though.

What Lazy Day represents to me is simply not doing much . . . or just do whatever you want. Take two hours today to do whatever the heck you want, or should I say, "Whatever the heck you FEEL like doing," because our choices we make daily, to work out and eat right or do something to better ourselves, are, after all, what we want! Today, however, you get to do things that may not be an instant cure for anything, but in the long run, you need days like this in your life every so often! Don't worry about the laundry. Be in your phone as much as you want, and don't worry about eating healthy (but hopefully you feel like it anyway). Postpone a call until tomorrow. Yes, put things off for one day. Whatever is on your mind that just has the smallest incline of stress attached to it, deal wit it later! Of course if you have a job, go ahead and go to work, but the rest of your day, be whoever you want to be and do whatever makes you feel relaxed and happy! And the most important part: Don't feel guilty for doing nothing. I know when you have goals and dreams, you constantly feel like you need to or have to do this and that. But guess what? We are doing many things to improve ourselves every day right? Take a day off because it will balance out your stress level, and as I said in my intro, pushing something to tomorrow (sometimes) can have great benefits for you — for your motivation, for your inspiration and for overall energy towards the goals you have! Relax.

Day 24

Pineapple Fried Rice

This recipe is another improvisation type recipe. The pineapple was suggested to me by my dear friend, Nicole! She made this dish worthy of a spot on my daily recipe list! I thought it was too boring before, but oh how my kids love this! And so do I!! We loved it before the pineapple was added, but my gosh, it makes it go from being yummy to YUMMMMMMMMMY! I smile while cooking this dish and I don't even mind standing by the stove the entire time making sure I stir enough for the rice to not get stuck on the bottom of the pan.

Prep: 5 min, Cook: 30 min, Total Time: 35 min

What you need (4 servings):
2 cups of rice-uncooked (brown or white)
2 cups of frozen, mixed veggies
4-6 strings of green onion
2 eggs
3 tablespoons of olive oil
1 can of tuna in water
1 (drained) can of pineapple (or a 3rd of a fresh pineapple)
Seasoning: Salt, Pepper, Paprika, Garlic powder
3 Tablespoons of Soy sauce

Prepare:
1. In a large pot, heat up 4 cups of water with 2 cups of rice in it. Once it starts boiling, turn to low heat immediately, and let simmer for 18-20 minutes (with a lid) until all water is resolved.
2. In a large pan, heat up the oil and sauté the green onion for one minute on medium-high heat.
3. Add rice into the pan and keep stirring it while it cooks for about 5min.
4. Add seasonings.
5. Add the frozen veggies and keep cooking on medium heat for another 3-4 minutes. Stir, and occasionally check to see if the bottom of pan is still greasy. if not, add another tablespoon of oil!
5. Add the eggs in the pan, cook for additional 3-4 minutes while stirring
6. Add the pineapple and cook for another 2 minutes on medium to low heat.
7. If you like it spicy, add sriracha or chili powder to your liking!

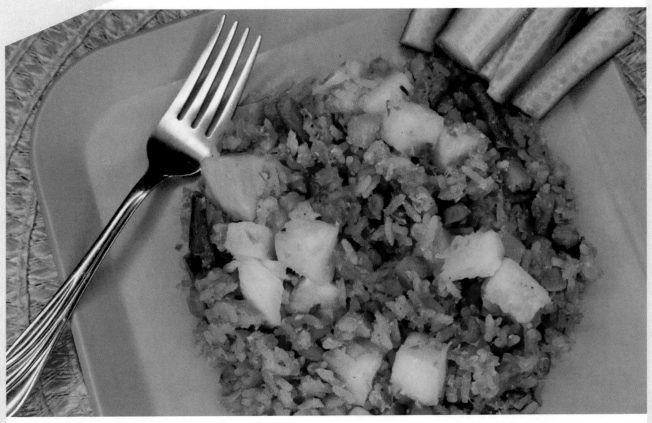

Day 24

Day 25

Yogi Day

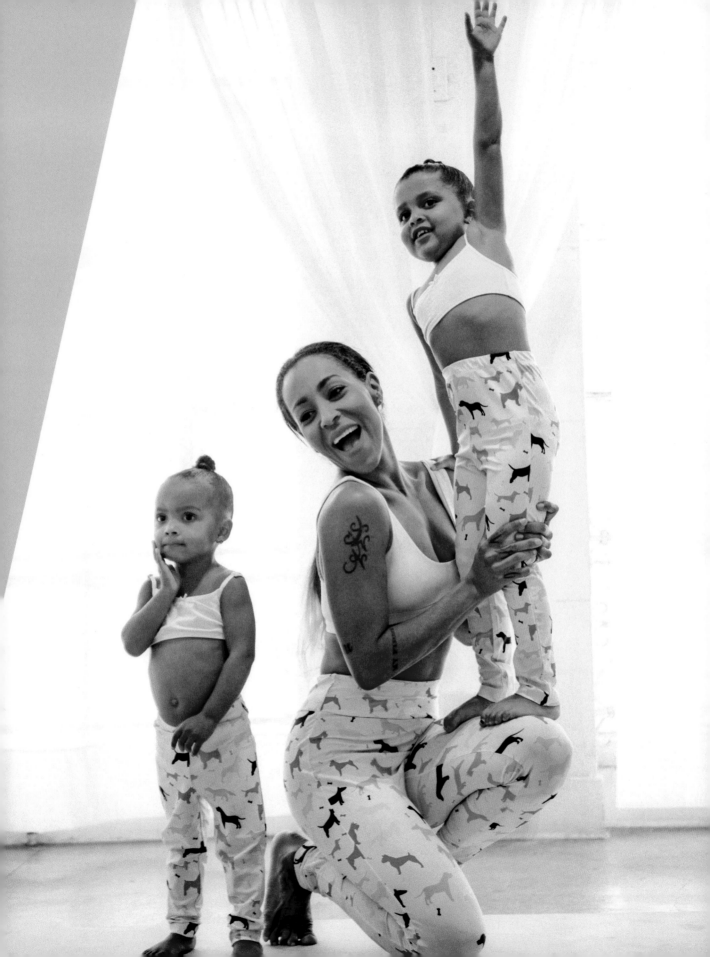

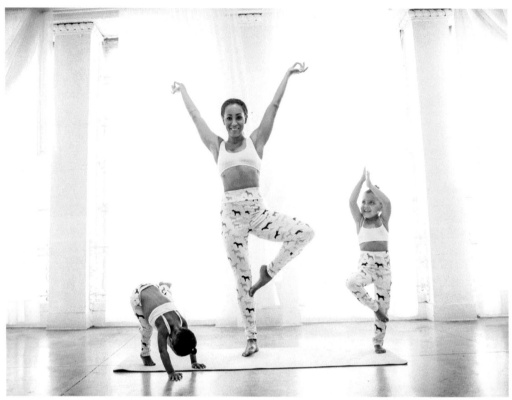

Something I've learned over the years from having to repeatedly get over certain painful events in my life, is that you must NOT dwell on the negative, the pain and the sufferings in life. Yes, you certainly should address those things, because shoving issues under the rug and ignoring pain is most definitely not a solution either, even when you give it time. There is a difference between addressing something and dwelling on it though. Addressing it means you're dealing with it while working on gaining control over the situation. Dwelling on it means you're continuing to let the situation control you without taking action to-

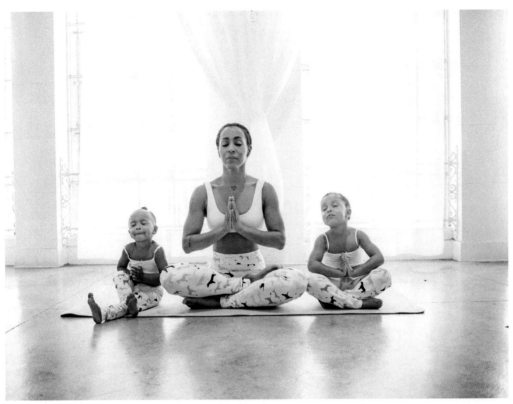

wards change. Through yoga you become more aware. And awareness of what's happening when you're going through something is of benefit for everyone involved — not just yourself.

And as if I haven't said the word "control" enough in this book, when you have control over your body, you learn how easy it is to have control over your mind and eventually, your life! And then, the magic begins!

Day 25

Ready for our Yoga Flow?

I'm going to jump right in since you know what it's all about now!!

How about trying it without going back to Day 5 and looking at the pictures? I want you to be in your own element. And remember, following doesn't matter: What matters is that you do each pose as best you can. Take your time with it, and don't rush through the flow. Challenge yourself to do it as slow as you can! Keep your mouth closed throughout the entire flow and breathe deep-

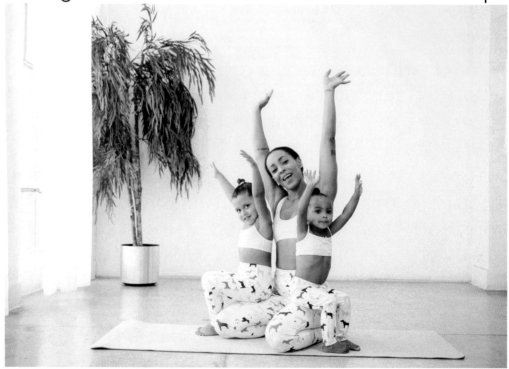

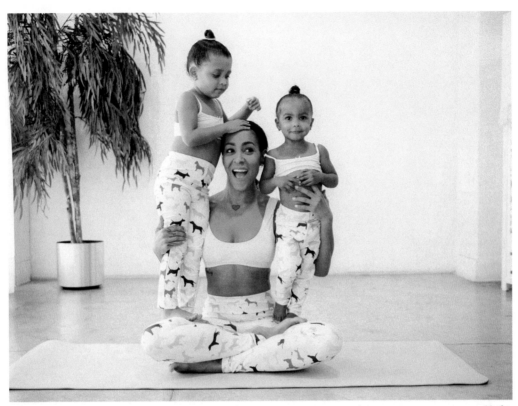

ly through your nose. By now you know: we call it Ujjayi breath.

Try to dedicate your practice towards something or someone today! It could even be towards yourself. It can be towards whatever it is that you are trying to change in your life. Let each breath be the power and the force behind the strength and courage you need to make these very changes. I feel powerful when I'm in a yoga pose. And as I addressed before, power in a yoga pose means it will be easier to apply power to my real life and its challenges.

Day 25

FOOD OF THE DAY

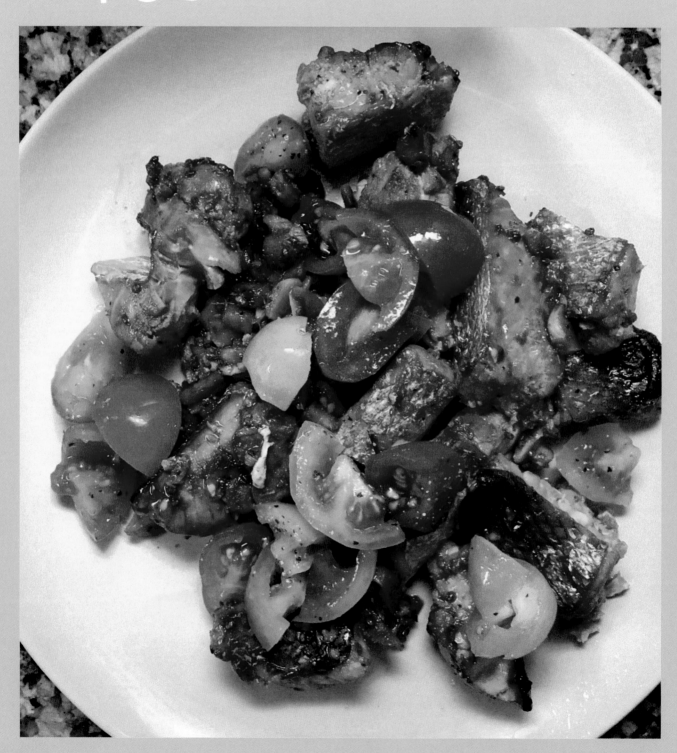

Just Salmon

I've tried making salmon many different ways, but this is probably one of the simplest, most yummy recipes. The only catch is that marinating takes about 30 minutes. Other than that, it's the quickest din din ever! And yes, you may add rice or quinoa or even bread on the side, but I like it best just by itself! Cutting carbs is made easy, because it really doesn't call for it. Enjoy!

Prep: 30 min, Cook: 7-10 min, Total Time: 40 min

Prepare:

1. Cut salmon into dices (about 2x2 inches).
2. Chop ginger (tiny pieces) and slice the garlic clove (thin slices).
3. In a bowl, mix the soy sauce and honey and add the garlic and ginger, then place the salmon cubes into the bowl and mix everything.
4. Let it marinate for 20-30 minutes (covered).
5. Heat oil in skillet (medium heat).
6. Place salmon into skillet and cook for 3-4 minutes, then turn and cook another 3 minutes. Make sure you use a non-stick pan here!
7. Sprinkle salt & pepper to your liking.
8. Serve on a plate adding tomatoes and sesame seeds.

What You Need (for 2 portions):

2 fresh 4 oz salmon filets
1 oz (4 inch fresh ginger)
2 garlic cloves chopped
3 tablespoons olive oil
3 tablespoons soy sauce
salt & pepper
8 petit medley tomatoes (cut into quarters)
1 teaspoon of honey
sesame seeds (optional)

Day 25

Day 26

Heavy Lifting

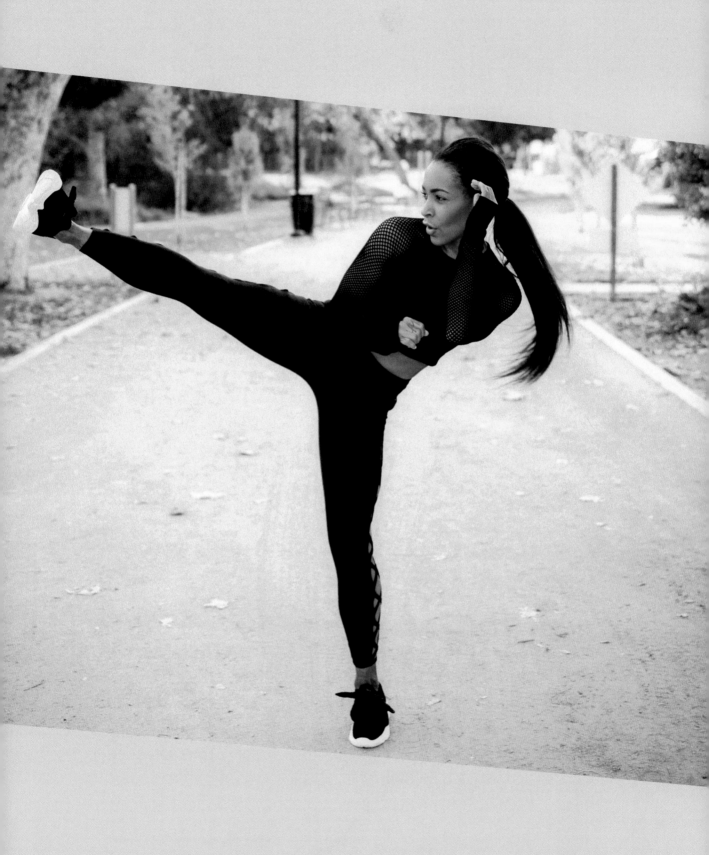

Hello, Beauty Queen! First things first! Let's get to work. On the agenda today is the workout from Day 13! If you have time to knock it out before anything else today, do that! It'll make your day so much better.

While the entity of this book is dedicated to us MOMS, I want to make today especially about MOTHERS. That's why I added another "Mommy" recipe, from *My* Mommy, that is. If you're not a mom, don't worry: This will still be good for you to read because you might be a future mom. However, if you don't desire to have kids, well, that is completely respectable. I once thought, "Having children is selfish," and even though I absolutely think having kids gives you such a better quality of life, I still believe it.

No one has kids for the kids. People have kids because *they* want kids usually. *They* want to be a parent, *they* want to better their life by adding to the family, *they* want to have someone to grow old with them and gain the experience of creating a life. Whatever the reason, we have kids for ourselves — so, that's what I mean by selfish. When we meet people and they ask about our life, one very common question is, "Do you want kids?" not "Do you want to make a kid happy?" Of course once they get here we want to give them the best life possible! And the selfishness, in most cases, vanishes. It often shifts to just wanting to be the best parent ever, which is great because that's the best benefit for the child. But the initial desire to have a child is to cater to your own desire and is all about *your* life. Sad, but true. Now, once they're here, you having moments of "If I didn't have the kids I could do X, Y and Z," or "Man, my social life is pretty much over," or even "I wish I could go back to when I was free."

These are all normal moments and there's nothing to feel guilty about. Being in the entertainment business and living in such a lively city as L.A., I get invited out multiple times a week. But almost 90 percent of the time I can't go because of my girls. But guess what? I'm okay with it. Good for me, I partied so much in my 20s and didn't have my first child until I was 31, so I almost feel like I've done and seen it all. So, what am I really missing? Not much.

From the many messages I get all the time, I'm aware that there are many younger moms who may feel overwhelmed by motherhood. One of the number one questions I get asked is how I do certain things with my kids around, and I mentioned (in my Intro) how to train your kids to behave while you're doing something for you. Now, I have to say this: When you have toddlers, like me, it only works for a small timeframe, but the key here is **CONSISTENCY**, and this is our word today. I get compliments on how

Day 26

well my girls behave all the time from   teach-ers, babysitters and just people who get to spend time around them. But the only reason my kids listen pretty well and recognize when they're wrong (and even make it right or apologize on their own) is because I made them understand that if they give me my moment, they're going to get reward-ed with something. Most of the time that reward is simply my time and devotion, because all my kids ever want is for me to play with them. They know, if they give me 20 minutes, their time will come — so they wait patiently. At first, yes, they may have tried interrupting me more, but I would ignore them (unless it was something urgent) until they got it. As a mom I always know when to tune in to their demands.

My girls also get a gift or some sweets every now and then for being good. If they keep mis-behaving, I use the common parenting method - Timeout - which works very well in my house. My youngest, Bronx, 2 ½ at the time of this writing, put herself on timeout the other day. I almost couldn't believe it. After I scolded her she went into her room and closed the door. She then waited five minutes, came back in the room where I was and said, "I'm super sorry mom." I could not believe it!

As far as working out while my kids run around, it wasn't always easy, but learning how to do you (while being attentive) is what makes it all possible. Like when I jump rope and Baby Bronx comes running into my space (and it happens often), I never mistakenly hit her with the rope. I have simply gotten good at multitasking, by practicing it — so it's natural when she joins me. Or I do my yoga flow and before I know it, the kids start climbing on top of me. Modification is my go-to in that moment. Hold a plank until they get bored and move on to their toys. It's not that hard. You just can't get discouraged. Keep at it and I promise you, as I said in Day 2, they will learn this is part of what mommy is and what mommy needs. They will eventually accept you and your space and understand if you keep at it and stay consistent with your work!!

Day 26

MOMMY'S LEEK PIE

The reason I decided to use this recipe in my book is because when I was about 10 years old, it was my favorite dish my mommy made! Healthy meets Indulgent, basically, and I never actually tried making it until I decided to write this book! I had to at least try making it once — just using my mom's recipe, for this book! It was so easy to make and tasted just like when my mom used to make it in 1993. My mother, at the time, worked at a place called "Reformhaus" which is a German retailer that specializes in healthy groceries free of synthetic preservatives and other health products. This dish was one of the most in-demand products, and my mom says she used to make three of these a day! She would then bring the leftovers home to us! I remember her coming home saying, "Ami Ich hab Lauch-Torte mit!" Translation: "Ami, I brought you Leek Pie!" I used to get so excited! The curry in this dish is what gives it that special taste! I hope you love it as much as I do!

Prep:10min. Bake:35min. Total Time:45min.

What You Need

(for a 9x9 inch pan):

2 pounds of fresh Leek
fluffy pastry (from cooler /not frozen)
2 eggs
1 cup of cream (substitute coconut milk for healthier option)
1 cup shredded cheese (of your choice)
1 tablespoon curry
olive Oil
nutmeg
salt & pepper

Prepare:

1. Place the fluffy pastry into the pan so it covers everything (even the sides).
2. Cut off the bottom part of the fresh leek and discard it, then wash it and chop it all up into about 1 inch rings.
3. In a pan, sauté the leek in 2-3 tablespoons of olive oil, add nutmeg, salt, pepper and ½ tablespoon of curry. Sauté for about 5 minutes on medium heat.
4. Put entirety of contents into baking pan with the pastry already in place.
5. Add shredded cheese on top so it covers the entire dish.
6. In a Bowl: Add Cream (or coconut milk), whisk the eggs, ½ tablespoon curry, salt and pepper into it.
7. Pour it over the cheese (it will spread and run all the way to the bottom of the pie.
8. Preheat oven to 350 degrees and bake for 35 minutes until cheese is golden Brown.

Let it cool of for a few minutes and enjoy warm or cold!

FOOD OF THE DAY

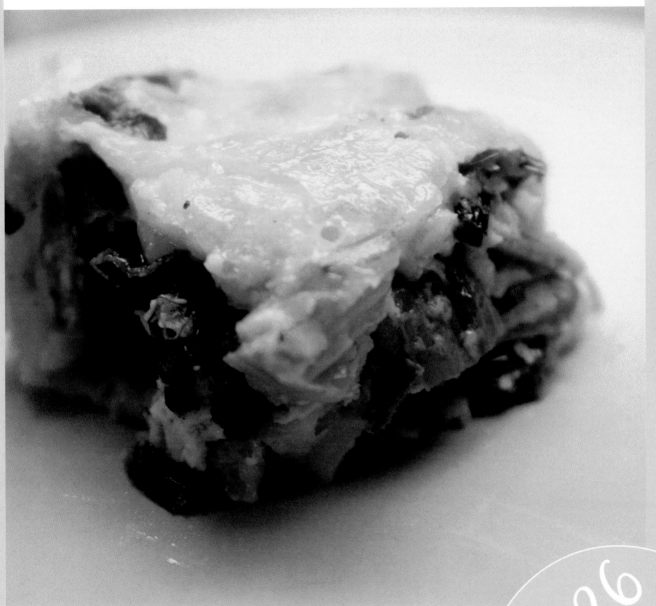

Day 26

Day 27

Meditate

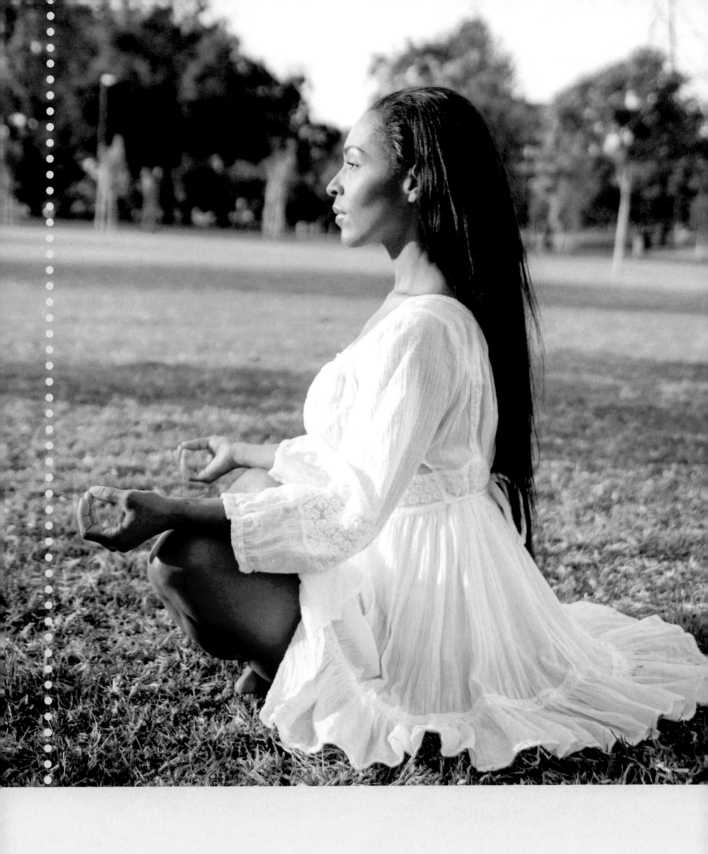

What do you think of when you hear the word meditation? Is it something you're curious about? Is it something you just don't know how to do or maybe feel that it's nonsense, or that it just doesn't work for you? Whatever it may be, meditating is proven to have great benefits for your life. It helps with anxiety, stress reduction, sleeping, focus, peace, attention span improvement, brain function and more. Honestly, the list goes on and on.

People have different ways of meditating. Generally, you'd think of sitting somewhere in silence with your eyes closed and just focusing on Being and Breathing, or another sensation within yourself, without getting distracted. My personal meditation journey started, again, when I got into yoga. Being that Bikram Yoga (my first experience among other yoga forms) is considered a "moving meditation," I learned how to get into a state of meditation I called "zoning out" while in class by shutting out any distractions from the outside world whenever I entered that yoga room. By doing that, I was able to balance my emotions and that was (and still is) such an amazing thing, since a lot of the time my days were ruled by emotions, even if I was trying to hide them. But even for someone who doesn't seem to be very emotional, meditation may be a useful thing to make time for! Much like I said on our Day 4 (Be Still), it is important to press "Pause" every now and then in our busy lives. We tend to rush through our days without taking a breather, and go from one thing to the next! A lot of the things I named on Day 4 are my way of meditating. I sometimes meditate in my car (when I don't have my kids) by turning off the music, driving in silence and not thinking about life's occurrences. I am that person who loves a long drive alone! I love taking road trips solo. I literally prefer that to having company.

Today's Task:

Try to be in a state of meditation for 30 minutes in whatever form you like. Similar to working out, where I said, "Don't think, just do," now. "Don't think, just BE."

Master the ability to completely relax physically and emotionally, which may not happen the first time or even the second time . . . but work on it. Try out different positions, preferably with a straight back! Be aware of your posture as well. No slouching on the couch! It is best to sit on the floor or if you're outdoors, sit on the grass.

Crossing your legs in front of you is a great posture to begin with. You'll then sit up straight and close your eyes. Try to be in the present moment and just BE. No negative thoughts and no drifting off think-

Day 27

ing about your To-Do list. Put your phone on silent. Mine is on silent so much that people get mad at me all the time for not answering or not responding right away. But guess what? Silence is sometimes good for my well being. 😉

If you have a hard time finding a quiet moment in the day, with non-stop mommy duties, meditate when your kids are in bed at night or even better, wake up 30 minutes early to meditate before beginning your day!

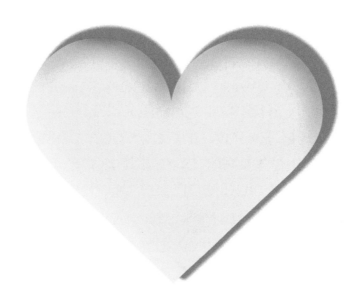

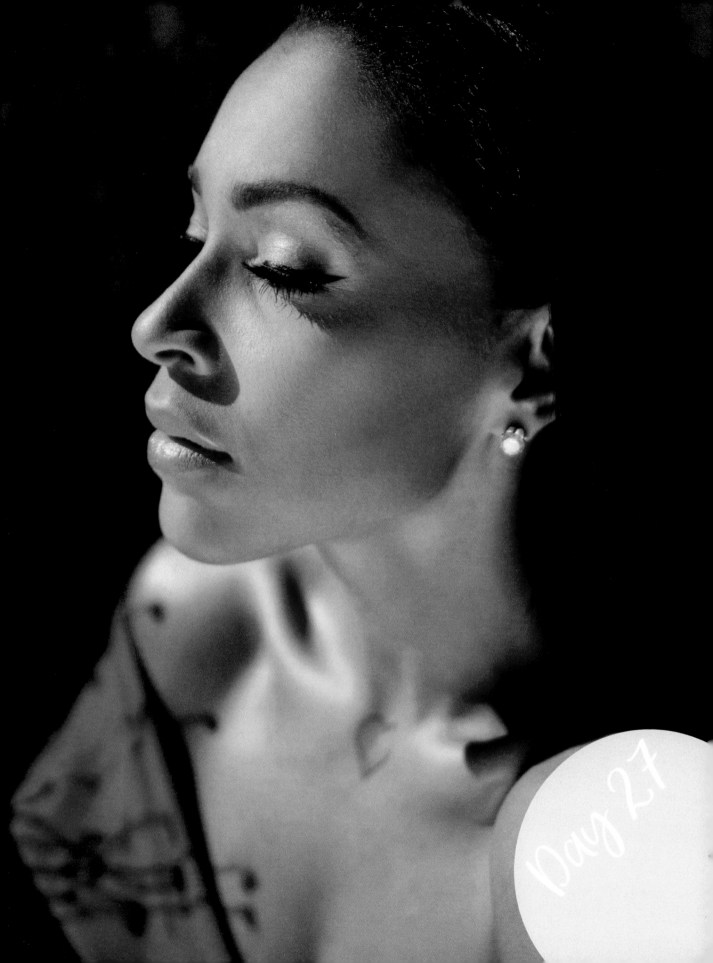

Day 27

Vegan Quinoa Broccoli Bowl

I'm not Vegan, however, most people that follow me know I love eating Vegan food every so often! First of all, it makes me feel better to consume less animal meat. Secondly, it is yummy and healthy! So why not skip the dairy and meat, even if you are someone like me, who eats EVERYTHING. Here's a dish I concocted (again). It came out so good the first time, and I didn't even really know what I was doing. I literally just mixed everything together and it was delicious!

Prep: 5 min, Cook: 15 min, Total Time: 20 min

What You need
(2 servings):

1 ½ cups of quinoa (uncooked)
½ of a small onion
2 garlic cloves (sliced)
6 oz broccoli florets
½ yellow, red or green pepper
2 Tablespoons olive oil
3 Tablespoons Soy Sauce
2-3 oz almond Butter
Salt and pepper

Prepare:

1. Cook quinoa in 3 cups of water. Start with high heat until it boils, then immediately set to low heat. Simmer for about 15 minutes until water is resolved. I like to add a teaspoon of salt for taste.
2. Chop up the onion into small pieces and slice the garlic (thin slices).
3. In a pan, heat the oil and sauté chopped onion and garlic for 1 minute (medium heat).
4. Add pepper and broccoli and cook for 5-6 minutes while stirring.
5. Add salt, pepper and soy sauce.
6. Add almond butter and continuously stir on medium-low heat until it is spread evenly!
7. Serve the broccoli and pepper mix over quinoa and enjoy hot.

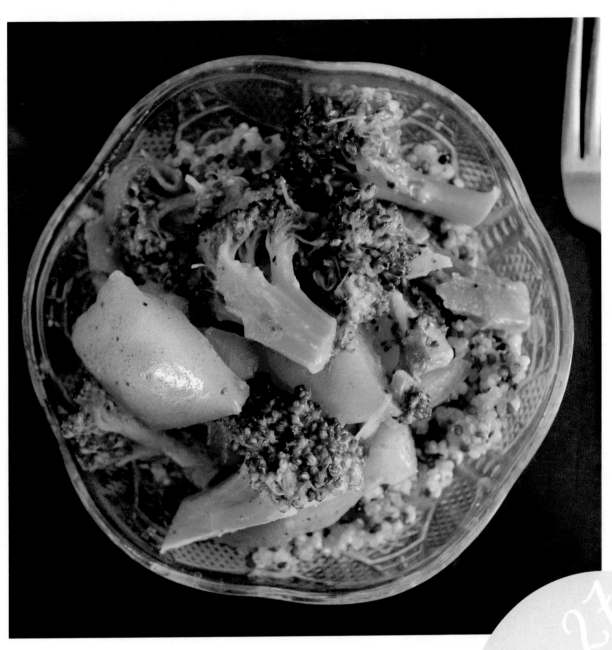

Day 27

Day 28

Write

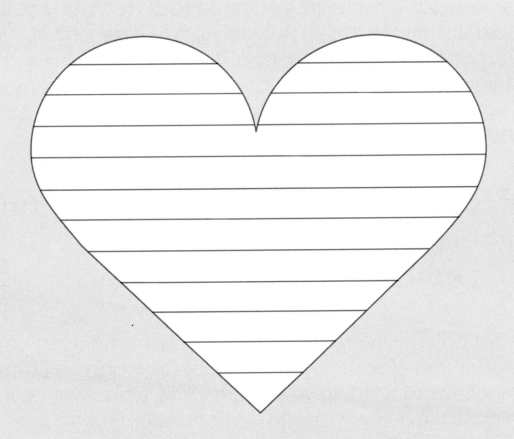

Many of us use writing as a form of therapy. I have done so much writing in my life that it comes kind of natural for me. However, I never thought I was a good enough writer to write a book, but hey, this is my second one, and I couldn't be more proud. I have come to the conclusion that when you doubt yourself, that's the moment you need to go for it, because the only thing that can happen is that it doesn't come out perfect or great, or it's a "fail," and people laugh at you. All of those things aren't tragic. The tragedy is if you do nothing when you have something to say. And here goes another one of my favorite quotes:

"It is better to create something that others criticize than to create nothing and criticize others!"

I believe every one of us has something to say. Even if you don't feel comfortable enough to share things, write it down. As long as you write from your heart, there is no wrong way. I consider writing art.

A little story: When I was 14 years old, I fell in love . . . or at least I thought I had fallen in love. As absurd as it was, it was with a stranger — a celebrity that I thought would be my only soulmate in this world. Ridiculous, I know, but this is what the 14-year-old me was doing. Don't laugh at me. This was a serious issue, which got me into writing. So there I was, 14 (with big dreams), and he was 17, and a big star. I couldn't tell nobody because who would believe that I loved someone I didn't know? NOBODY.

In hindsight, of course, I didn't love the guy, but the thing that mattered is this: I felt alone because nobody understood me. I lived in this imaginary world of myself and him by writing in a diary/journal, in the form of letters. Every night at bedtime I would write about my fears, my struggles, my insecurities and my loneliness. This little diary of mine (I still have it, by the way) saved me. It could have been to anybody — not just the guy I thought I loved. And that is my point here: It wasn't about who I was writing to, it was *that* I was writing to help myself cope with this "situation" I *thought* I was in, or that I was in, because to me it was real. I wrote a lot of things in my diary/journal because I felt my thoughts were safe there. No one was going to judge my truths or the things I felt. No one in the outside world would understand, but in my diary, where I was freely expressing myself, I felt like I was heard. Even to this day no one has ever read it (at least I haven't shared and probably never will).

Moral of the story, writing down something that bothers you can be freeing.

Day 28

Task: Write as if you were telling a non-judging soul. And yes, you may have told your bestie or sister or whoever is closest to you already, but dig deep. Everyone has something they haven't shared. And we all have something that worries us about the future. We are trying to eliminate worrying, remember. No, this will not take all challenges and concerns away automatically, but it will help you to deal with them.

As a matter of fact, I was open with you. Now how about you write to me. Here is your space:

Dear Amina . . .

_____

_____

_____

_____

_____

_____

_____

_____

_____

Golden Tea
(Tumeric-Ginger-Thyme)

You may also call it Health Tea! Turmeric is an anti-inflammatory spice, which also promotes cardiovascular health, balances cholesterol levels, supports weight loss, speeds up metabolism and promotes brain health, among other things. Combining it with the ginger and adding thyme which both of these are immune system boosters. This is simply just as the title says: "GOLDEN."

Prep: 2 Min, Cook: 13 Min, Total Time: 15 Min

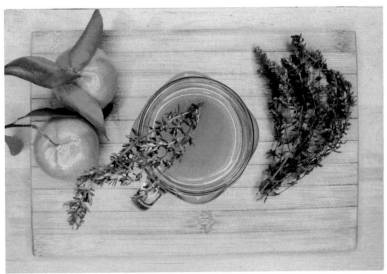

What you need
(for 4 cups):

2 teaspoons of turmeric (powder)
½ teaspoon thyme
2 oz of fresh (chopped) ginger
5 cups of water
Honey for sweetening

Prepare

1. Place everything in a pot (heat on high) until it boils. Immediately turn the heat to low and let it simmer for 13 minutes.
2. Serve in cups and add honey to your liking.
3. Add a fresh squeezed orange for an amazing taste twist.   (Optional)

Day 29

Wear Yourself Out

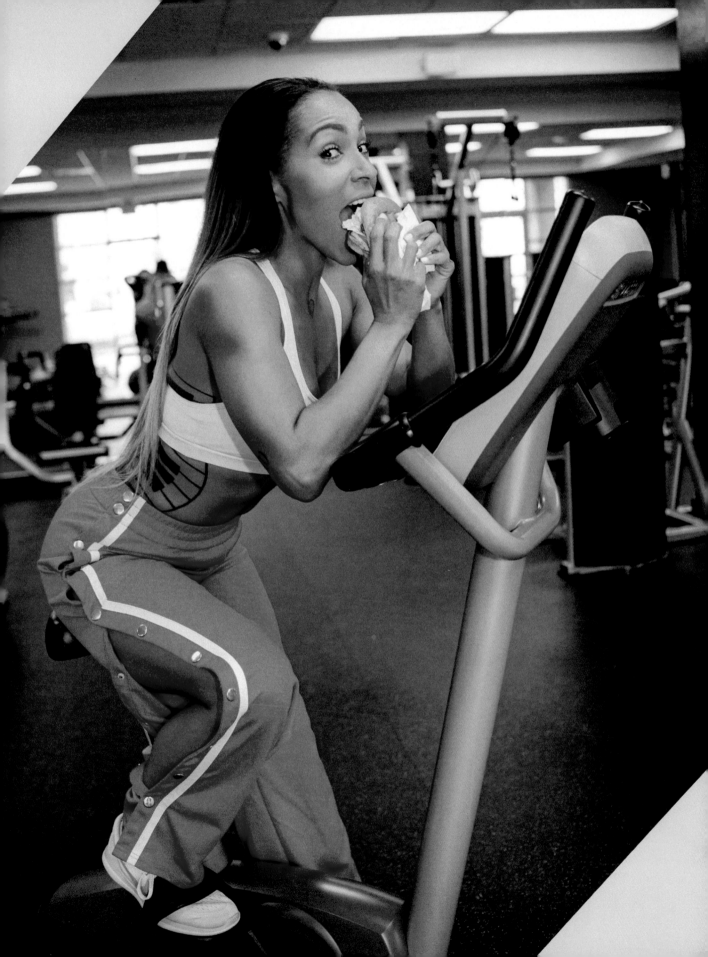

thing I can do is accept that I didn't speak. And here we go full circle again, about the time I talked about dwelling on something.

The harder things to accept are those things you have to accept for good, like disappointment from a friend. Work on acceptance and it gets easier. I used to have such a hard time accepting things in my life, especially about myself. It was a big part of why I wasn't happy. The things I could change, I worked on changing. The things I couldn't change, I worked on accepting.

Now, it almost comes easy to do both — making changes and accepting things that are out of my control, and I am so much happier.

If you run outdoors, make sure you keep the 2 minutes on, 2 minutes off pattern, and just run as fast as you can run for 2 min. straight each time. Don't take it easy here: Push through!!! YOU GOT IT!

You will be feeling like a warrior after this workout. You can switch the order and do your cardio first, which is what I always do because I like it less! Get it out of the way!

Today's Word: ACCEPTANCE

I almost got a tattoo of the word Acceptance once. It has become such a big and important word in my life. These days, I remind myself probably a few times a day, to accept certain things that bother me. And when you fully do, life is better! Yes, obviously I am talking about the things that you aren't able to change right away. right away, like when my skin breaks out and I feel horrible. Yes, I can do something about it for the long run, but today, nothing will change. I'm going to look just like I am! Accept it. Move on.

Or it could be that I haven't had time to clean before leaving the house, and it's a huge mess. Yes, I can take care of it later, but right now, it is and will be messy until I get to it. Accept it! Or I might say, "Man, I should have spoken to the guy at work today about my idea. I missed my chance." Well, too late now, so the only

262

And the Days keep coming back! The days we must push ourselves, that is! Think of it more like you're earning your "Feel Good" points. Each time you workout hard you get rewarded with a dose of happiness, because remember: Feeling Good = Happiness. Another thing to remember is that the stronger you get physically, the lighter you'll feel. Something like a push-up, which you might hate doing, can actually become fun just like a hand-stand, which one might think of as just a cool thing to master, but it has really become a fun activity with benefits. Win, Win, Hooray. For those who hate working out, you can get there with a positive mind and with consistency, just like everything else in life!

Today's Workout:

Abs and Arm Exercises from Day 9!

Plus, a 20 minute run, 2 minutes on, 2 minutes off!

Beginner: ON: 6, Off: 3

Intermediate: ON: 7.5, Off: 3.8

Advanced: 8.5, Off:4

Garlic Brussel Sprouts & Sweet Potato Wedges

This really could be a side dish, but I personally love to have this as my meal. And I don't even miss my meat or protein. For instance, if I eat this for lunch, I'll just have a higher protein dinner or visa versa. I may even just have some protein snacks throughout the day to balance it all out. Brussel sprouts are not everyone's favorite, but I promise you, it's all in the seasoning and in the art of not overcooking, so they maintain a nutty flavor! Try it and see for yourself.

Prep:10 min, Cook:30 min, Total Time: 40 min

Prepare:

1. Set the oven to 400.
2. Peel the potatoes and trim the ends of Brussel sprouts, then rinse everything
3. Cut the sprouts in halves and slice the potatoes in about 2 inch, wide stripes.
4. Place everything into a bowl and mix with the oil, salt and pepper and garlic.
5. Spread it onto baking sheet and bake for 15 minutes, then turn over and continue baking for another 15 minutes.
6. We are trying to achieve a slight crisp for both the sprouts and the potatoes, so make sure you check after 30 minuses of baking. If need be, add some more minutes until everything is golden brown!

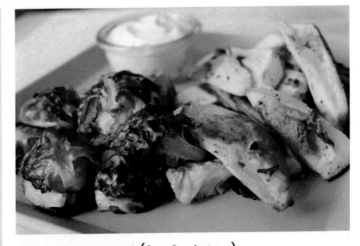

What you need (for 2 plates):
½ lb fresh Brussel sprouts
3 large sweet potatoes
3 cloves of garlic (minced)
2 Tablespoons of Olive Oil
salt and pepper
¼ cup of grated
parmesan cheese

YUMMMM!

Day 29

Day 30

Celebrate!

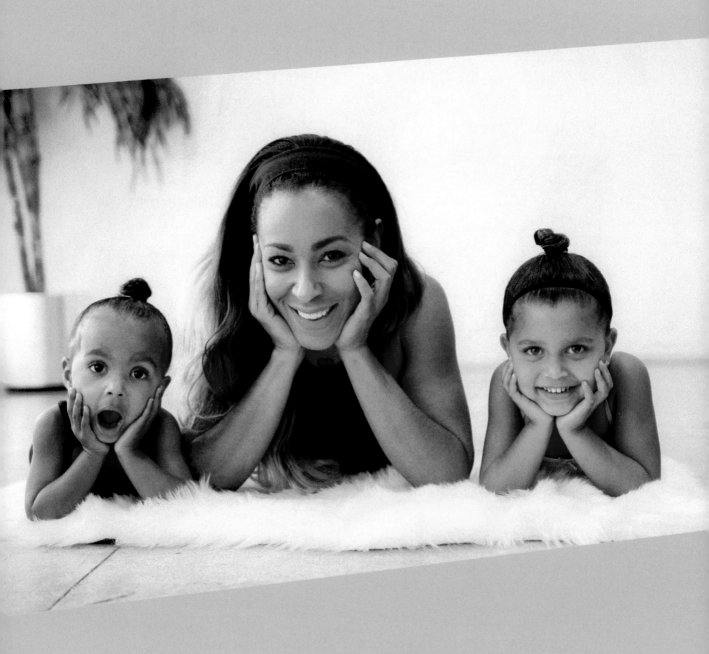

We did it! YOU did it! Being that it ain't new to me (to just Do It), let's keep the focus on the amazing YOU! I'd officially love to welcome you to MI Health Family! This was only the beginning to what will hopefully be a permanent change. Better yet; this will lead to Permanent Changes in your daily life.

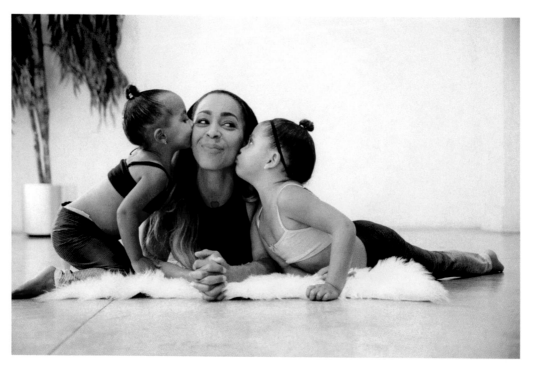

Now, if we could only celebrate together, wouldn't that be cool? Today is Celebration Day. How do I celebrate? Simply by doing all of what I love doing! Maybe even calling up some friends to come over, get lots of food, some wine, make cocktails at home, or if I have the option, get a babysitter and go out for some fun! If you celebrate by having a Lazy Day, go ahead! It's whatever you like! If you celebrate by having the most intense workout of your month, go ahead!! It does not matter and there aren't any rules.

BE You, BE Free, BE Happy, BE Healthy which I'm hoping you feel you're at least on your way to Becoming!

Today's Word:

Kindness!

Love yourself and love others. Hate is weak, but love is strong! Be Kind at all times, and especially be kind to yourself! When you aren't feeling something, it may not need to be vocalized. Yes, if it's someone close to you, always let them know how you feel, but in a nice way! Speaking your true feelings and giving your opinions to your friends in a nice way is absolutely fine, and even necessary. But NEVER act out if you catch yourself in a moment where you want to tell a stranger something other than kind words. That only reflects back on you in a negative way.

Day 30

MI Skinny Watermelon Margarita

     I don't make drinks at home a lot, but on a day like today, it is a fun addition to any meal and a great way to create a celebratory atmosphere in your own home! Obviously, if you don't drink alcohol (good for you!), this will not be for you and my suggestion is repeating one of the other 30 recipes in this book. Maybe the one you've enjoyed the most is a great idea. I chose a margarita because it's so easy to limit the ingredients here and make it a low calorie drink! Besides that, it is just super refreshing.

DRINK OF THE DAY:

What you need (for 1 cocktail):
1 oz tequila (of your choice)
4 tablespoons of fresh squeezed lime juice
1 tablespoon of orange juice (not from concentrate)
2 tablespoons of club soda
2 teaspoons of Agave nectar
¼ cup of diced watermelon
ice cubes
1 tablespoon salt (optional)
cocktail shaker (optional)

Prepare:
1. Slice a lime and go around the edge of your glass rim with it.
2. Place salt on a small plate and dip your glass into it for salt rim.
3. Mix all ingredients into the glass (or shaker if applicable).

CHEERS!!

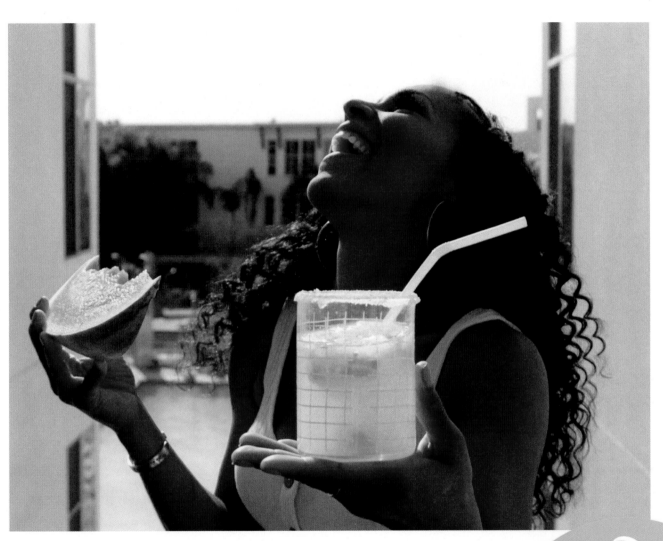

Day 30

Made in the USA
Middletown, DE
18 September 2019